# When Older Is Wiser

A GUIDE TO HEALTH CARE DECISIONS

FOR OLDER ADULTS AND

THEIR FAMILIES

# When Older Is Wiser

## A GUIDE TO HEALTH CARE DECISIONS FOR OLDER ADULTS AND THEIR FAMILIES

Patricia Parsons, B.N., M.Sc.
Arthur Parsons, M.D.

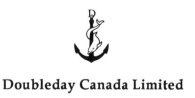

Doubleday Canada Limited

This book is dedicated to Gwen and Bill Houlihan and Marjorie and Max Parsons, our parents.

The case stories in this book do not represent any specific individuals or circumstances. These composites have been created by the authors from a variety of experiences during their health care careers.

**Canadian Cataloguing in Publication Data**

Parsons, Patricia Houlihan
When older is wiser: a guide to health care decisions for older adults and their families

Includes bibliographical references
ISBN 0-385-25427-X

1. Aged — Medical care. 1. Parsons, Arthur H.
(Arthur Hedley), 1943-  II. Title

HV1451.P3 1993    362.I'989/   C93-094201-9

Cover illustration by Helen D'Souza
Cover design by Avril Orloff
Printed and bound in the USA

Published in Canada by
Doubleday Canada Limited
105 Bond Street
Toronto, Ontario
M5B 1Y3

# Contents

# When You're Sixty-four

**W**HAT DO George Burns, Sophia Loren, Pierre Elliott Trudeau, Queen Elizabeth and Mother Teresa have in common? It may not be the first characteristic that springs to mind, but they are all old, at least by the usual standards. Why is it that we don't think of them as old, while others we know of the same chronological age seem to be old above all else?

Perhaps the answer is that these people are in control of their lives and making decisions for themselves. They continue to do the work they like, and they make useful contributions to society.

What about you? Are you old — or do you think you are?

These days "old" is a very imprecise word. You might start to feel old because of arthritis in your forties; or you might be in your seventies already with no physical complaints and sharp as the proverbial tack.

This book is for you if you are old enough to know better: old enough to take charge, and old enough to think ahead. You may already be retired — or just dreaming about it; or you may be seeing what modern life is like for older people through the experience of your parents.

There's no doubt that the modern age has brought us longer lives — a blessing to some, a burden to others. But modernity has also brought the belief in individual rights and autonomy.

In the health care field, this translates into a decrease in the "Father knows best" attitude so many of us have been subjected to by doctors. With less paternalism from our caregivers, we not only can but must make more of our own decisions about complex health care issues.

Why not see this new empowerment as an opportunity to plan for your later life? With the help of this book, you can educate yourself about modern health care, explore your feelings about aging and take control by bringing these feelings into the open and discussing your wishes with caregivers and family members.

This book will help you to make a number of important decisions about your future, such as:

- Do I need to change family doctors now to get the kind of care I want later on?

- Do I want my family closely involved in my health care, or do I prefer to be independent of them?

- What kind of nursing home would I find acceptable?

- Under what circumstances would extending my life be more important to me than the quality of my life?

- How much medical intervention would I tolerate during a critical or terminal illness?

■ Am I willing to take risks or make sacrifices for the sake of others?

These are difficult decisions. But delaying them won't make them any easier. Start now to give yourself as much time as possible to make good choices.

As health professionals, communicators and aging baby boomers ourselves, we have written this book to give you the knowledge and the tools you will need to take control and keep control in your inevitable encounters with modern health care. You may feel young and healthy at this moment. But if you were to suffer a stroke tonight, leaving you unable to express yourself, do you know what measures you would want taken? More important, do your relatives and doctors know?

Perhaps you are already faced with having to make decisions for someone else; if so, you have probably said to yourself, "I wish I knew what Mother wanted." This book will help you with that dilemma and will encourage you to take steps so that you do not leave your own children in the same difficult position.

You may not consider yourself old, but we are all moving in that same direction, like it or not. Wouldn't it be comforting to know that getting older means becoming wiser, too?

# PART ONE

# Understanding the Essentials

# 1 : Everyone Gets Old

*"Grow old along with me*
*The best is yet to be*
*The last of life for which the first was made."*

**W**ITH THE EYE AND PEN of the poet, Robert Browning surely had a more romantic notion of what it means to grow old than do many of the baby boomers of the 1990s. We look toward our twilight years and take on the mantle of battle. "I will not grow old, I will not grow old!" seems to be the cry. Well, this is one battle we will lose: *everyone* gets old.

Aging is really not an illness any more than pregnancy is. But it does place us at greater risk of having our bodies break down, thus forcing us into ever more interactions with the medical system. Never has this been more true than today.

At the start of this century, people died young of diseases that are now preventable or curable. Physicians then could not cure disease; they could only treat the symptoms of illnesses such as pneumonia, rheumatic fever and measles, common killers of children and young adults in the early 1900s.

Today it is rare indeed for these diseases to be fatal, and many acute illnesses that strike adults in mid-life, such as gastric ulcers and Hodgkin's disease, are curable too. With improvements in lifestyle, we have greatly reduced the toll of heart disease, once a frequent killer of adults.

The dark side of this form of progress, however, is that most of us would probably rather die from a sudden illness or heart attack, given the choice. Instead, modern medicine has decreased our chances of having this relatively quick and painless death and has increased our chances of living through a long, painful, chronic illness before reaching the end, which may itself be laboured and unnatural.

Life expectancy has increased by about twenty-eight years since 1900. But medical science, which has so greatly contributed to this increase, has made little progress in preventing, let alone curing, the debilitating diseases of aging such as arthritis, stroke, Parkinson's disease and Alzheimer's disease. For some, those "extra" twenty-eight years will be plagued by disability, institutionalization and even dementia.

A middle-aged man today can expect to live, on average, to his mid-seventies; a middle-aged woman to her early eighties. At present about 12 percent of the North American population is over sixty-five, and that percentage is growing. There has been a tripling in the number of centenarians, those who live to 100, over the past twenty years.

Will the greater numbers of older adults change society's overall attitude toward aging? If this is to happen, there are some formidable barriers to overcome.

## AGEISM IN NORTH AMERICA

With the baby boom soon to turn into the "geezer boom," as *Newsweek* memorably dubbed it, will the sheer numbers of older people change the prejudicial way that older people are treated?

Ageism has been compared to racism. People make assumptions about the capabilities and potential contributions of individuals based on their chronological age. Mandatory retirement has been pointed to as a blatant example of discrimination on the basis of age, and the phenomenon doesn't seem to be receding.

Most of us have little sense of what it is like to be old in North America today until we experience it ourselves. But one young person has been there — and back. She may be the only young woman who has direct knowledge of how an eighty-five-year-old woman is treated in our society.

In 1979, Pat Moore, then a twenty-six-year-old industrial engineer from New York, embarked upon a two-year odyssey that took her to 116 cities across the United States and Canada. Using make-up and specially constructed prosthetics, she transformed herself into an octogenarian. She made a point of seeking experiences that she could undertake both as an old woman and as a young woman. She would ask a store clerk for help in purchasing something in her aged disguise, for instance, then return the next day as her attractive young self and compare the response of the same clerk.

What Pat Moore found was terrifying for those of us who have yet to experience old age. As she related

9

in her 1985 book *Disguised: A True Story*, she was treated with everything from simple disdain to violence; at one point in her project, she was severely beaten. She concluded that elderly people are usually treated with anything but respect, and that ageism is all too common.

In health care, the issue of discrimination based on age takes on a slightly different complexion. Here's a common situation.

Pierre J., a healthy seventy-year-old, has always looked after himself. He continues to be active doing volunteer work in his community and lives a happy life. As a result of a viral infection, Pierre has now developed end-stage liver failure, for which the only treatment is a liver transplant. The medical center to which he is referred doesn't have a hard and fast maximum age for transplant recipients, but it has never transplanted a liver into a recipient over sixty.

At the same time, Thomas S. is admitted to the same hospital, also in liver failure. At forty-two, Thomas is an apparently recovering alcoholic. In all other respects he and Pierre are equally qualified for a transplant. Do you think that Pierre will be given equal consideration in the recipient selection process? Chances are he will not, and the reason will be his age.

Health professionals cannot be completely blind to a patient's age, for many valid medical reasons. But is age-related discrimination justified in *all* situations? Both you, as an older individual, and the health care system as a whole must consider the proper role of age in decisions about your health care. We will return to this question in later chapters.

## AGE SEGREGATION

Society's attitudes toward older people are also influenced by a number of recent changes in family structure.

There was a time when the extended family was the norm in North America: members of several generations had regular contact and perhaps even shared a home. Older parents took an active part in the lives of their children and grandchildren. Young children were accustomed to seeing people two generations older as often as they saw their parents and siblings. In general, homes and society were not segregated by age.

Several social factors have joined to break up the extended family. One of the most important is the itinerant nature of society today. It is very likely that you moved away from home to go to college or university and, upon graduation, chose not to return to your home town, either to look for greener pastures or to find any pasture at all that would hire you. The economy has certainly had an impact here. As a result, the geographical gulf between family members can be immense.

The old model of father at work, mother at home caring for children is no longer reliable. Facts of our lives like divorce, working mothers, and child-rearing postponed or forgone altogether have affected today's older generation and will affect tomorrow's even more. Today a woman who must work outside the home finds it difficult to care for aging parents; tomorrow the same woman may have no grown children nearby to care for her. Those baby boomers who

11

remained childless, enjoying their double-income-no-kids lifestyle, may look around and see little support to see them through.

Today's answer seems to be that older people who do not have families to care for them should be cared for in homes or residences specifically designed for them, resulting in what some people regard as ghetto-like segregation by age. With a decrease in the opportunities for interaction between the generations, the younger generation — including young health professionals — is growing up with no real knowledge of how to interact with its elders.

## QUALITY VERSUS QUANTITY OF LIFE

As you age, you will find this crucial question arising in many forms and various contexts: Is it important to you to live a high-quality life even at the expense of a long life?

Your answer to this question will influence decisions about your health care. Furthermore, it is an important philosophical question to ask your own doctor or any other health professional who might be involved in your health care in the future. If your views are in conflict with those of your caregivers or even those of your family, you may be facing an uphill battle to control your own health care as you age.

One of the basic ethical principles that have guided the decisions of health professionals for centuries is "sanctity of life." This concept is based on the idea that human life is sacred and should be preserved. In health care this principle requires the health professional, first and foremost, to do everything in his or her power to preserve human life.

Belief in the sanctity of life is part of the mindset of many practitioners who have graduated and continue to graduate from medical schools. Many physicians, both young and old, believe that life, however it is defined, should be preserved at all costs and that any available treatment measure should be tried. They see it as their duty to give care and save lives. Medicine is a war, and death is the enemy.

Patients often have a different view. Many people believe, especially as we age, that life is more than a beating heart and a set of breathing lungs. The quality of life, which can only be measured subjectively, is often more important to people than its length. For one person, a good-quality life might mean simply the ability to eat, bathe and get dressed without help; another person may need much more. Each of us has to make that judgment.

Deborah F. is a sixty-year-old widow, the mother of three grown children. She was diagnosed with Alzheimer's disease at age fifty-two and for several years has lived a comfortable but supervised life with one of her daughters and the daughter's young family. A lover of reading, cooking, knitting and bridge, she was able to continue these pursuits until recently. But in the past two years she has begun to show the usual signs of mental and physical deterioration that are common with advancing Alzheimer's disease.

When Deborah was diagnosed, she read all she could find on the disease and became well aware of what probably lay ahead; she discussed the future with her daughter. Deborah realized that she would eventually not be able to do the things she loved and that at some point she would fail to recognize even her own grandchildren and would require physical care.

She has told her daughter that she does not want anything but supportive care in these later stages of the disease. She has asked her daughter, who will be making some of her decisions for her when she no longer can, not to allow any aggressive treatment of any acute medical problem that might arise. Deborah has decided that, for her, the quality of her life is more important than the length of her life.

Kenneth L. is also sixty. His wife, six years his junior, is a nurse who continues to work. Six months ago he was diagnosed with terminal cancer of the lung, and he knows he will die soon. With deteriorating health and increasing pain, Kenneth knows he has to make a decision about whether to allow the doctors to treat the pneumonia for which he has just been admitted to hospital. If he chooses palliative treatment only, the objective of his care will be to make him as comfortable as possible, and he knows that his life will probably be shortened. That care, however, will put an end to his constant misery.

Although Kenneth is bedridden and unable to care for himself, and although every day is a reminder of all that he can no longer do, he wants to see his granddaughter graduate from university. She will be the first in the family to do so, and he knows that for his wife, the experience will be that much more satisfying if he is there to share it. He chooses aggressive treatment, thus deciding that, at least for now, quantity of life is more important for him than quality.

Clearly, in each of these cases, the individual involved is the best person to make the decision. No one else deciding for that person, whether a family member or a physician, could know exactly what he or she wants, unless they have discussed the possibilities together earlier. The choice between quantity and quality is not an issue for older adults only, but it is likely to affect you to a greater degree than it does young people.

Robert Browning's view of aging was romantic indeed. Sophocles, poetic in his own way, took a more practical approach: "The immortal gods alone have neither age nor death! All other things almighty time disquiets."

Perhaps we can keep control and not let time get away with everything.

# 2 The Genie of Modern Medicine

In a hundred years, as humankind approaches the turn of another century, there is little doubt that historians will look back on the twentieth century as one of enormous innovation in science. One of the sciences that will stand out above the crowd will be medical science. It is hard to imagine that the advances of medicine in the twenty-first century will come even close to the progress we have made since the Victorian era. How much more medical sophistication can we cope with?

One urban folk tale, told and retold and even published in a number of medical journals, makes an important point about modern medical technology. The story takes place in the intensive care unit of a large urban hospital. In this unit was a patient who was on a heart monitor. One morning, just as the doctor was about to make rounds, he noticed that the monitor at the nursing station did not seem to be working properly. He immediately called the biomedical engineering department and asked them to send someone up to fix it. The technician quickly arrived on the unit and began the laborious process of searching for the origin of the problem. Starting at the wall receptacle where the bank of monitors was plugged in, he worked back toward the patient's bedside. All connections seemed to be in order. Finally, when no one could find any technological problem, they examined the patient and found the origin of the monitor's failure to show the patient's heartbeat. He was dead.

True or not, this tale points out one of the traps that we can fall into when faced with an array of technologically sophisticated medical equipment. When overused, the machines begin to control us and we lose the ability to relate to one another as living, breathing human beings. The machines seem to come between us. As consumers of health care services, we can't let that happen.

It's worth keeping in mind, too, that all medical treatments, whether high-technology or not so high-tech, carry risks as well as benefits. A simple arthritis drug, for example, could result in stomach ulcers in a small number of patients. This is what doctors call "iatrogenic" disease, a condition that is actually caused by medical treatment.

With the aging process, these risks increase. Many treatments affect our bodies differently in later years than they did while we were younger, often causing more side effects. And as medicine grows in complexity, its risks multiply accordingly. Many of the newest procedures are not even tested on older adults, so their precise effects may be unknown.

## THE MARVELS OF MODERN MEDICINE

Whatever else it has also done, modern medical technology has increased the length of our lives and, to a degree, the quality of those lives. No longer do we commonly die in North America from simple problems like appendicitis, pneumonia or kidney failure. Following decades of research and development, health professionals can apply their new knowledge and use the latest tools of their trade to provide us with care. An abundance of available tools encompass diagnostics (defining the problem) as well as therapeutics (treating the problem).

We have antibiotics to fight off almost every manner of infection, cancer chemotherapy drugs to pulverize some cancerous tumors, CT scans and MRIs to give us three-dimensional pictures of the insides of our bodies, organ transplants to replace our failed organs, artificial ventilators to breathe for us when we cannot, infusion pumps to count the drips of the intravenous solution so that the nurses don't have to, electronic thermometers, dialysis machines, heart-lung machines, artificial joints — the list goes on and on. This is truly a marvelous time to be sick. Or is it?

One of the persistent failings of medical technology that are of special concern to us as we age is that while great strides have been made in the treatment and prevention of many acute illnesses of the young and the middle-aged, there is little to offer sufferers of chronic illnesses that are a significant risk to older people. There are no cures nor even adequate treatments for these illnesses that affect the quality of our lives.

Already great numbers of people suffer from arthritis, Parkinson's disease, Alzheimer's disease, osteoporosis, chronic obstructive lung disease and other debilitating diseases that get progressively worse as we age. And as the number of older people in our population increases, the number of people who suffer from these long-term problems gets larger. We continue to await breakthroughs in these low-profile but increasingly prevalent diseases. As Dr. Rosemary Hutchison says, writing about what she calls the new "high-tech chronic" patient, "The genie of modern technology has not lived up to its promises."

High-technology care is not the answer to every medical problem, but its prominence in modern North American health care forces us to make important decisions when faced with both technological and non-technological choices. We need never be forced, however gently, into accepting the high-tech solution to every health problem we face. We would do well to remember in all these discussions what Aristotle said: "Education is the best provision for old age."

## THE GENIE HAS ESCAPED: WHAT NOW?

Many health professionals are beginning to realize that our emphasis on scientific achievements has had a negative effect on the humanistic side of health care. At least to a degree, the media must be held accountable for the interest in high-tech health care. On one level, it's understandable. If you were a reporter concerned about ratings of your television news show, which topic would you be more likely to write about: Alzheimer's disease or transplantation of baboon hearts into humans? Experience shows us that most reporters would choose the transplant story because of its more sensational nature. But the truth is that far more viewers will be able to relate directly to a story on caring for Alzheimer's patients than will ever have need of a heart transplant of any kind.

There have been four general effects of letting this genie out of its bottle:

- a decreased emphasis on the "art" of medicine;
- a view of the sick person as a broken machine;
- increased costs of health and illness care;
- a steadily increasing number of medical specialties with consequent complications in health care delivery.

You may be surprised to see medicine described as an art. Hippocrates, the father of medicine, wrote sometime around 400 B.C. that "medicine is the most distinguished of all the arts." Art, by its very nature, involves human characteristics such as the application of creativity, intuition, empathy and emotional self-discovery, all of which seem to be useful attributes for health professionals to possess.

The modern truth has been, however, that these personal qualities have been overlooked when medical schools have evaluated applications of aspiring doctors. For many years, the single-minded emphasis on mastery of the basic sciences in pre-medical education has resulted in undervaluing the human

21

side of medicine. Some North American medical schools are beginning to rethink the relative merits of arts versus sciences for their future doctors, but we will be left, for many years to come, with the legacy of medical practitioners who were educated to believe in the supremacy of science. This has played no small part in medicine's current reliance on quick fixes.

A second effect of the thirst for technology has been an altered view of sick people. Instead of seeing the patient as a person, the high-tech practitioner sees the patient as a broken machine. Perhaps we can learn something from practitioners of traditional Chinese medicine. Unlike their counterparts here in the West, they view the human body not as a machine but as a garden. Gardens cannot be "fixed" as you would fix a broken car engine; they must be nurtured.

Considering that the Chinese have been successfully viewing medicine this way for twenty-three centuries, they must be doing something right. The current Western tradition puts the health professional squarely in the role of mechanic, which changes dramatically the relationship with you, the patient. As the authors of *The Healing Arts* have said, "Perhaps the greatest loss that medicine has suffered over the course of the centuries is that of personal contact."

The third effect of all this medical technological innovation has been an increase in the costs of providing health care. This is becoming such a problem in North America that we are now looking at how best to allocate these scarce resources. While there are other factors involved in these growing costs, technology is certainly an important one. Even the way we pay health care personnel indicates that we value highly the more technological approaches to care. For example, nurses who work in intensive care units receive a higher salary than do nurses who work in palliative care with terminally ill people. This wage gap persists although it seems absurd to compare the work done by the nurse assigned to one patient in the intensive care unit with the work of the nurse in charge of ten people, one of whom she may assist to a peaceful death during her shift.

It is estimated that health care spending in the U.S. is over $900 billion annually and in Canada, it is over $64 billion; costs are rising in both countries. The rate of spending growth is outstripping the annual population growth rate, and there is little indication that higher costs have resulted in significantly better health. About 40 percent of all health care spending is on people over sixty-five, and an increasingly large proportion of this money is spent on people in the last weeks and months of their lives.

In many cases terminally ill patients, old and young alike, have their lives extended by modern machines and drugs, sometimes with questionable quality of life. Placing the elderly patient with incurable congestive heart failure on an artificial ventilator in the intensive care unit might extend that life for a short time, if you define life in very minimal terms. Viewing it from another perspective, all we are doing is extending the dying process without providing this individual with any more "life" at all.

Finally, a fourth consequence of the increased use of medical technology is the increase in the number of medical and allied health subspecialties. This has only added to the complexity of an already complicated system. Almost every time a new discovery is made in medical technology, we witness the birth of either a new medical specialty or a new group of allied health professionals. Before the advent of ultrasound technology, for example, there were no ultrasound technologists, just as before the arrival of open heart surgery and dialysis machines, we didn't have health professionals called perfusionists. And these are but two examples of an ever-growing list of disciplines.

Statistics from the early 1980s indicated that there were well over 5 million Americans employed in health careers, in over 700 different occupational areas. Clearly, the health care industry is a growth area in employment. In Canada, the two industries predicted to have the largest growth by the turn of the century are physicians' services and medical laboratories and hospitals.

All this change and diversity in health care results in even more confusion for the patient who is trying to sort out who's who.

Especially in large, urban teaching hospitals, the array of personnel can be very daunting. When you awake in the morning you come face to face with your "nurse," but is that person a registered nurse, a nursing assistant, a licensed practical nurse, a student nurse, the nursing instructor or the head nurse? You may still be sorting out the nursing staff when a group of assorted doctor-types arrives. It becomes even more difficult for you to be heard among all the learned opinions about what is best for you.

Knowing who does what is extremely important if you are going to decide what kind of health care is best for you and who is the best professional to provide it to you. If the price tag of the service isn't a factor for you, then not even your budget can help you decide (and it isn't a particularly good way to make decisions regarding your health care anyway). Should you go to a chiropractor or an orthopedic surgeon? Should you go to a physiatrist (a medical specialist in rehabilitative medicine) or an occupational therapist? Can a nurse practitioner help you? The only way you can decide is to keep on top of what is happening, by reading about new developments in health care and asking lots of questions.

## MEDICAL TECHNOLOGY AND AGING

People of all ages can be overwhelmed and dehumanized by medical technology. But health professionals take special considerations when deciding whether to apply technological approaches to older patients, and you need to be aware of their thoughts on the subject.

As suggested in chapter 1, a patient's age is a significant factor in the decision to apply or not apply technological resources when there are not enough to go around. When both could benefit from it, professionals must choose which patient should get the ICU bed: the forty-year-old heart patient, or the seventy-five-year-old heart patient.

Health care personnel struggle with such dilemmas almost every day of their professional lives. The irony is that caregivers often decide to "save" patients who might well have preferred to slip away — but because patients have not thought about such eventualities or have not communicated their wishes, the ethical, moral and medical struggles of all involved end in an outcome that no one wanted. The older patient who is comfortable with bypassing the ICU in favour of a younger patient would save the workers from needless deliberation, if only they knew. The informed older patient who can see the bigger picture will understand if the health care workers decide to give the bed to the younger patient, all things being equal.

Even when resources are adequate, practitioners of high-technology medical care as well as of low-technology care must know when to stop. Dr. Nancy Jecker of the University of Washington has written: "Only the physician who understands natural limits and uses this understanding to set wise boundaries avoids the error of excessive confidence." A doctor who doesn't know when to stop doesn't know either his or her own limits or the limits of modern medicine. There is something almost egotistical about a physician who seems to think that if he or she just did that one thing more control over life and death could be achieved.

This notion of natural limits is not a new one in medicine. As long ago as the fifth century B.C., physicians of the Hippocratic tradition saw that they needed to be aware of the limitations of their art. The individual who can play the most important role in the difficult decision to stop, however, is the patient. As a patient you have a responsibility to help health professionals give up the quest for the "cure" in every situation and to help them see that death is not always the enemy.

Is it even possible for modern health care to return to its person-centered approach of the past? Is it possible that the disease-orientation of some caregivers might be altered to see the person at the heart of the problem? If the less beneficial trends of modern medicine are to be turned back, it will be because health care consumers become aware of what is happening and exercise this knowledge in practical ways to assist in the delivery of their own health care.

# 3 : Allies
and
Well-wishers

GEORGE BERNARD SHAW had some very interesting perspectives on the relationship between doctors and their patients. He said: "I do not know a single thoughtful and well-informed person who does not feel that the tragedy of illness at present is that it delivers you helplessly into the hands of a profession which you deeply mistrust." Although he was writing in the early twentieth century, he could just as easily have been forecasting late-twentieth-century beliefs. Indeed, the cornerstone of the relationship we have with our health caregivers ought to be trust, but we do not always know enough about their work to be able to give them our confidence.

Caregivers and family members alike have a role to play in your health care decisions, and this involvement tends to increase over the years. First, then, you need to be aware of who's who in the "health team" and examine the factors that affect the decision-making of each of those caregivers. You need to examine especially your relationship with your family doctor and determine how the power position of the physician may cause you to make decisions that might not be in keeping with your own value systems.

Then there is your family. Are your loved ones entitled to have a say in your health care decisions as you age? Do they have a right to know your most intimate medical problems? And which ones should play a part? Examine your relationships with important family members and consider their role in your health care.

## WHO'S WHO ON THE TEAM

Trust ought to be the cornerstone of your relationship with your doctor and other caregivers. But one important component of modern health care often makes it difficult for this trust to develop. This feature of the system is commonly called the "health team" approach to care.

The "health team" concept arises from the great expansion and specialization of health services that we have already discussed in chapter 2. Doctors, nurses and other health professionals form the "team" that provides care for each individual patient. This approach has both good features and bad features for you, the patient. The down side can become increasingly apparent as you get older and relinquish some of the control of your decision-making to younger family members and caregivers.

If you are hospitalized for something as seemingly simple as varicose vein surgery, you might expect to be cared for by a vascular surgeon; a number of nurses who specialize in areas like operating room assistance, recovery room care and post-operative surgical care; and an anesthesiologist. A reasonable enough team; but if you develop a complication, such as a blood clot in your lung, the expansion of the team will be rapid.

You immediately find yourself in the Diagnostic Imaging Department (once called the X-ray Department, but there are now many other ways to diagnose you other than old-fashioned X-rays), where a nuclear medicine technician is assigned to complete your lung scan. When you return to your room you are confined to bed, where an IV nurse (the one with the long needle who will put an intravenous catheter in your arm) is waiting for you. Before the day is over, you are visited by several other doctors in training and a respiratory technologist. Your team has become considerably more complicated. On the whole it seems like a very good thing that there are health professionals who are able to give this kind of specialized care, and that there is a team organization to coordinate their comings and goings.

With any kind of team, however, there are problems. These may affect both the care that you receive and your ability to make your own decisions about that care.

First, while you may be unaware of it, the health team is probably suffering from what can only be described as turf wars. Doctors are concerned that nurse practitioners are encroaching on their areas of responsibility; registered nurses fear that nursing assistants, licensed practical nurses and others such as health educators are invading their territory. And these are only two groups concerned about their practice areas. These interprofessional wars and disagreements can leave the patient in the middle, not knowing who to turn to for advice and assistance or whose opinion to believe.

The second peculiarity of the team, which is sometimes related to turf wars, is the kind and extent of communication that exists between members. When the members respect one another, the communication is usually good, and differing points of view are welcomed and listened to. Each health professional, by virtue of his or her personal background and professional training, will view a situation differently. This is often an advantage to you as a patient, since differing points of view help you to see all angles. But, on the other hand, if you are not armed with enough independent information beforehand, different perspectives are likely to become confusing to you.

How can you know whether a team has good communication? Listen to what your doctor, for example, is saying about the nurses, and to what the nurses are saying about the doctors, technicians, dietitians and others. And further, listen to *how* it is being said. Watch the interaction between members and consider the kind of relationship that is apparent. Do they talk to one another, or does one doctor talk while everyone else listens? Do they seem genial with one another? Are they personable with you or coldly clinical? If their communication among themselves is faulty, then their communication with you will probably be faulty as well.

You may wonder who will speak up for the older

patient in this team structure. An advocate, someone who has your best interests in mind and who will plead your case in an educated way, can be very important in health care. With the complexity of modern medicine, it is difficult for you to know everything that you would like to know, even with a diligent effort.

The person who can probably advocate best for the patient is the family doctor. If you have developed a relationship with a personal physician over time, then he or she is probably in the best position to understand both your perspective and the requirements of the system.

When you are in hospital, you may have another resource. Many hospitals today have patient advocates. While the person in this position may often feel like the complaints department, listening to litanies of criticisms about everything from the food to the television reception, there is a much more useful role that he or she can play. It is this person's responsibility to plead your case should you or your family need help in being heard by the doctors or nurses. The patient advocate has no say in medical decision-making but may be able to make the health care personnel aware that you need to play a bigger role in issues that affect you.

Your health team may all have your best interests in mind and still find they disagree about the best and most appropriate approach for your care; these disagreements are not uncommon. Remember that each individual health care worker comes into the situation with his or her own set of personal values. As much as medical, nursing and allied health schools today try to teach ethics and ethical decision-making to their students, they cannot change those basic values.

Values, the important beliefs that guide our lives and our decisions, develop as the result of a combination of many things, including our family relationships, cultural and racial backgrounds, religious upbringing, personal experiences and the whole spectrum of what touches us as persons. Essentially, *anything* that touches your life may play a part in determining what you hold to be important. No one's personal values are ever quite the same as another's, and each health professional is an individual who is likely to view each situation from his or her own perspective. This will almost certainly affect the advice they will give you.

For example, if you are faced with a decision about whether you will accept a particular treatment, a nurse or doctor who has faced a similar situation, perhaps with a family member, is unlikely to be completely objective in giving you guidance. Although that kind of identification with the problems of the patient is frowned upon, it is a human frailty.

One final thought about the health care team approach: although each team member has a valuable role to play, it is often difficult to decide who can and cannot be trusted when you don't have time to develop anything but a superficial relationship with any of them. For you to be able to trust all of these people, it is necessary that you have faith, at least to some extent, in the system of health care within which they work.

Consider what happens when the cautious traveler plans a trip. He calls his travel agent to book seats on an airline that is reputable. He has used this travel agent before and has some faith in her recommendations. Before leaving for the airport, he checks the weather forecast and then heads out. Upon boarding the plane he pays attention to the safety demonstration and checks the location of the exits. At some point, he will have to sit back and trust that the pilots have made good decisions and have done their best. The worried passenger cannot go into the cockpit and begin to ask numerous questions about fuel and safety checks. Most passengers do not have enough basic knowledge to do so anyway.

Dr. Franz Ingelfinger, former editor of *The New England Journal of Medicine*, one of the world's most prestigious medical journals, has this to say about faith in physicians: "I do not want to be in the position of a shopper at the Casbah who negotiates and haggles with the physician about what is best. I want to believe that my physician is acting under higher moral principles and intellectual powers than a used-car salesman." On the other hand, Ingelfinger believes that a doctor who merely gives the patient choices and tells the patient to choose independently is shirking his or her duty to recommend a course of action after presentation of the pros and cons of the alternatives.

The best way for you to cultivate some trust and faith is to ask all your questions and do your research and to think, in advance, about a variety of possible health care scenarios that might involve you as you age. If and when one of these scenarios finally does face you in reality, you may be ready.

## THEY'RE ONLY HUMAN

This may come as a great surprise to those who grew up during the era when physicians and other health professionals occupied a somewhat elevated state in our society. Doctors have fallen off their pedestals. Several social trends have contributed to this state of affairs but none so much as the realization that doctors are only human. This is rather ironic in an age when much of what doctors are capable of doing resembles acts of God.

Aldous Huxley said, "Experience is not what happens to a man, it is what a man does with what happens to him." This is particularly true of how the life, medical care and educational experiences of one human doctor will shape him or her. Various doctors and other health professionals might describe the same patient's illness, probable outcome and best treatment choices quite differently, each putting a unique slant on it. A family doctor may consider the whole patient and the effects on the patient's family; the medical specialist may see only the affected body system; the nurse may consider only the nursing needs.

Doctors, like the rest of us, are affected by fears and needs. Two current social trends are especially likely to play on those emotions and to influence an individual doctor's decision-making and advice to you, the patient. One trend is the alarming increase in litigation against doctors. The other is the way we pay for medical care.

During the past decade, lawsuits against physicians and hospitals have multiplied. One has only to read the daily newspapers to see the evidence. It's far from clear that doctors and other health professionals are actually more negligent than they used to be, but just the possibility of being accused of negligence can change a doctor's attitude.

Imagine your family doctor has a friend across town who has just been slapped with a malpractice suit because she failed to order a very sophisticated medical test for an elderly patient who subsequently died. Although she contends that there was no reason to perform this test and that it would probably have had little effect on the eventual outcome, the grieving family charges that her lack of action may have contributed to their mother's death. Now your doctor is seated across from you and is trying to be objective in advising you about a similar test. Despite the fact that you may not need it, he may be scared enough of being in the same position as his friend that he wants to protect himself from a possible suit. He fills out the requisition and makes your appointment.

Your doctor's decision is not unnatural, from his perspective. One of the realities of medical and hospital practice in the 1990s is that patients often arrive in medical offices on the offensive. They are armed with the media's interpretation of the latest developments in leading-edge technology, and they demand equal access as a consumer's right. This is a far cry from the days when the doctor called all the shots.

The combination of litigiousness and patient demand has caused many doctors to be defensive and overly cautious, to the point of overusing the system. A frank and open discussion of all the pros and cons, with full awareness of your doctor's concerns, will yield the best decision.

The other important human factor in your doctor's decision-making framework, whether he admits it or not, is a result of the North American fee-for-service structure of medical care. Regardless of whether the fee is coming from the government, from an insurance company or out of the patient's pocket, a fee for a particular service will come the doctor's way.

For example, there are four possible ways to treat your gall bladder disease: classic surgery; lithotripsy (using shock waves to pulverize the stones) if available; endoscopically removing stones (through a scope passed down into the stomach and into the small intestine); or laparoscopic surgery (removal of the gall bladder through two little stab-like incisions). Your family doctor has sent you to a surgeon who can do the classic surgery to remove the gall bladder but cannot do the other procedures. The surgery will probably solve your problem, and the surgeon will get paid for it if you decide to proceed. If you opt for any of the other approaches instead, the surgeon will have to refer you on to someone else. There is obviously a possibility that this knowledge will affect how and even sometimes if he will explain your options to you. Although this may seem unethical from your standpoint, this surgeon knows that he can help you with your problem and may not even be aware that he is approaching his explanation of your options in a biased way. It has often been said that if you are holding a hammer, everything looks like a nail.

What can you do if you think that your doctor is presenting a biased recommendation? If you are uncomfortable, start by specifically asking the doctor if there are any alternative approaches. The doctor may present these in a biased way as well, but at least you will know more about where you stand. If you are still unhappy, seek a second opinion, or go back to your trusted family doctor, who probably sent you to the consultant in the first place, and ask for a more educated opinion than your gut feeling.

## THE POWER PROBLEM

The traditional doctor-patient relationship has always been characterized by lopsidedness. The physician has held the position of power, because the patient goes to the doctor in a time of need and the physician uses his or her greater knowledge and skills to meet that need. In many respects this imbalance of power is appropriate, but after years in a relatively exalted position, doctors can fall prey to an unhealthy attitude that affects their decision-making. This attitude is what medical ethics textbooks call paternalism.

Derived from the Latin meaning father, paternalism is loosely defined as approaching patient care with the attitude that the doctor knows best and will decide what is right for the patient. Although most doctors do know a great deal and do have the best interests of the patient at heart, no doctor can know precisely how you, the individual patient, will feel about any given issue. Other than providing you with the best possible medical information and advice, a health professional has no more right than any other person to decide what is right for you. But paternalism turns perfectly good caregivers into do-gooders.

You might think that the health professional will recognize the older patient as a source of wisdom, but this is not the case. Often older patients are treated like children, as if they had lost their ability to be fully functioning adults. This can be seen in small ways every day in our hospitals. When an elderly patient does not respond well, doctors and nurses are often quick to relate the lack of response to any one of a number of age-related conditions; only later do they realize that the silent shock they observe is the dignified reaction of a seventy-six-year-old woman who has never been called by her first name by her juniors. The use of first names is only one way that health professionals may fail to show respect for older patients. As the age gap between older patients and younger health professionals widens, lack of respect is likely to become a more frequent problem.

While health professionals need to be more aware of their tendencies toward paternalism, you the patient need to speak up for yourself when you sense a lack of respect. There is nothing at all wrong with saying to your doctor or nurse, "I prefer to be called Mrs. Bell."

## YOUR RELATIONSHIP WITH YOUR OWN DOCTOR

Doctor-patient relationships are paradoxical. On the one hand, doctors are told that they need to be more human in their encounters with patients. On the other, they must maintain what is called a professional distance. Finding a balance between the two can be difficult for health professionals, but if you understand this, you can help to shape the relationship that is best for you. When you are able to sustain a good, trusting relationship with a family doctor, you have a significant ally in decisions you will inevitably have to make about your health as you age.

Many older adults — perhaps as many as 90 percent of those over sixty-five — do not have a family physician. One reason is that earlier in life you probably chose a personal physician your age or older, and that doctor will eventually either retire or die. Developing another relationship with a doctor may seem to be more trouble than it is worth but it is, indeed, worth it. Don't wait until a crisis is upon you to find a new family doctor.

In all likelihood your new doctor will be considerably younger than you. You may have already experienced the shock of the generation gap. It can be quite unnerving at the age of forty or fifty, when you still consider yourself to be quite young, to walk into the office of the doctor who has taken over from your family physician for summer vacation, to find that this person looks like he is hardly out of high school. It's not just the young look of the face. It is also the earring in one ear, the denim shirt and the way he calls you "Ma'am."

This is one of the many changes you will have to get used to. It is likely that, as you get older and are faced with the health care system more frequently, many of the doctors, nurses and others who will care for you will have considerably less life experience than you do. It may seem peculiar to share some of your most intimate concerns with or even place your life in the hands of individuals who are as young as and even younger than your own children.

On its own, a doctor's relative youth should not be a barrier to a good relationship with you. But beware of the family doctor — young or not so young — whose heart is simply not in caring for older people. Many caregivers find this part of the family practice frustrating. Their feeling stems directly from the medical school mindset of the quest for the cure. The need to prove oneself more powerful than either disease or death may overwhelm a medical practitioner when faced with elderly patients who suffer from a variety of chronic illnesses and who are obviously closer to death than are younger patients. In fact, some medical practitioners who specialize in geriatric medicine estimate that people over sixty-five suffer from an average of three to four chronic disorders such as diabetes, arthritis, osteoporosis and arteriosclerosis. This fact itself can be offputting to some doctors.

What you need to know is how your current doctor or a doctor you are considering feels about treatment for older adults. The only way for you to find out about this is to ask him or her, preferably before you are actually much older yourself. Although it might be nice if you could remain with the same doctor for your later years, the family doctor who enjoyed seeing you through obstetrics and caring for your young family may not derive the same satisfaction from older patients. This doctor will probably not be the best choice to support you as you are faced with health care decisions.

What should you look for in choosing a family doctor who will be supportive of you as you age? Some of the following qualities might help:

- a doctor who shares your value system regarding the quality versus the length of life;

- a doctor who treats you with the level of respect that you require in a professional-patient relationship;

- a doctor who patiently answers all the questions that you want answered about any issue that affects your health care;

- a doctor who is able to be honest about any limitations he or she might have regarding your wishes for your future care;

- a doctor who stays actively involved in your care even if you require referral to a specialist of one kind or another.

Developing a trusting relationship with a caregiver now could be one of the most important aspects of taking charge of your health care decisions as you age. This trusted ally will be able to mediate between you and the system, or even between you and that other set of potential do-gooders: your family.

## BUT THEY MEAN WELL...

There is no doubt that our family members can and do play very important and valuable parts in our health care, but defining the limits of that responsibility can often be difficult. Family members can provide much-needed emotional support when you are faced with a difficult medical problem; and they can provide physical care of varying levels, from reinforcing healthy lifestyle choices to assisting in recuperation from illness, depending upon your relationship and their resources.

This, however, is often not the extent of their involvement. If your relationships are open and honest and health care issues and preferences have been previously discussed, their knowledge of you can help you to sort things out. On the other hand, if the relationships are not quite so healthy they may take it upon themselves without being asked to decide what is right for you in a given situation. Family members have been known to decide that Mother shouldn't be told about her terminal cancer, in spite of the fact that Mother has never said that she doesn't want to be told. The limits of your family's involvement, then, need to be determined before problems arise. Include your family in the decisions you will make as you read through this book.

There are many people in our lives who will play a part in decision-making about our health care. It is a good thing that we are not alone in these decisions, but the role that each plays needs to be sorted out long before the need for their input arises.

# PART TWO

# Controlling Your Health Care

# 4 Your Right to Decide

HEALTH PROFESSIONALS rely on a number of principles when they must make choices in their practice. Although there is no absolutely right or wrong decision when the question relates to morality, these principles can provide a foundation for necessary choices that, at the very least, can be defended.

You will find that some of these same principles can be applied to your own decision-making. From your point of view as a patient, these principles will revolve, to a great extent, around the exercising of your rights.

Your most important right in this context is your right to decide for yourself. Understanding that right will help you deal with the inevitable obstacles to your decision-making, obstacles that become increasingly troublesome as you age.

## EXERCISING YOUR RIGHTS

It seems that the topic of rights appears almost daily in the media. We hear about human rights, women's rights, consumer rights, the right to die, the right to life — and the list goes on. One of the more recent additions to this list is patients' rights.

47

Individual rights are claims that we make on others and on society; more than that, they are *justified* claims. Your right to a fair trial, for example, is justified by law. Your moral rights, however, are a bit more difficult to identify and agree upon, because not everyone in North American society shares the same morality or justifies the same claims. You, as the holder of the right to decide for yourself, need to remember three things about this right, which professionals call autonomy:

- You cannot be forced to exercise this right; you choose to exercise it or not.

- Because health professionals have agreed that you should be allowed to make your own decisions under most circumstances, it has become a justified claim and they have a duty to uphold your right.

- You cannot exercise this right if whatever you believe you have a right to is unavailable to you in a particular circumstance. You cannot exercise your right to choose to have a heart transplant for your heart disease if there are no hearts available.

As described here, in the calm, abstract language of ethics, it is hard to imagine anyone disputing your right to decide for yourself. But in real life your rights can come into painful conflict with the needs and wishes of others.

Maria G. is a widowed seventy-three-year-old retired nurse who worked until she turned sixty-five and has been relatively healthy all her life. Although she has become a bit forgetful over the past couple of years, she has lived very independently, maintaining her own apartment. Two months ago, while bathing, she discovered a lump in her right breast. She has not told anyone yet. She knows that this is very important information for her daughter to know for her own future health, but she also needs time to consider what she will do before she is bombarded with what she knows will be well-meaning advice.

When Maria finally does tell her family doctor, he immediately sets the wheels in motion for all the diagnostic tests necessary to determine whether she has cancer. She agrees to the tests because she knows that her daughter and her granddaughter will need to know if they are at increased risk of developing breast cancer. But she has read everything that she could find on breast cancer treatment and survival, she has spoken with a representative of her local Cancer society and her family doctor, and she has already made up her mind what she does and does not want. She agrees to the minor surgery to remove the lump, but that is the extent of the bodily invasion that she wishes. Finally, the diagnosis is made and breast cancer is confirmed.

Maria sits down with her daughter Gina and very calmly and rationally discusses her decision. Gina is now bordering on hysteria at the thought of losing her mother. She cannot comprehend why her mother does not wish extensive treatment. Maria realizes that Gina, thirty-five, does not understand her point of view, because she is seeing it through the eyes of a distraught daughter who refuses to give up her mother and who has much of her life yet to live. As a nurse, Maria has seen many women, young and old alike, face the devastating news of cancer, and she has watched the outcome of the treatment. Knowing all this, she has made her decision.

When she is visiting with her grandchildren one Saturday, Maria overhears Gina and a friend discussing Gina's tentative plans to have her declared incompetent so that Gina will be able to give consent to more rigorous treatment. Rage is Maria's first reaction, and then she is frightened.

This hypothetical case is more real than we would like it to be. Many people believe that they are making decisions in another person's best interests, but that notion of "best interest" is a very subjective one indeed. Each of us has different reasons for making particular decisions for ourselves.

## AUTONOMY AND THE HEALTH PROFESSIONAL

Health professionals have been taught the importance of upholding their patients' autonomy. But it can be particularly difficult for health professionals to respect this right because they believe that they know what is in a patient's best interests.

What's more, health professionals learn two overriding principles that are supposed to govern the care they provide: the commitment to "do good" and its corollary "do no harm." After all the time they have spent learning their art and their science, they should be in a good position to give advice that is designed to "do good." And what is "good" for the patient is obviously what is "not harmful." Thus, in an effort to uphold their own ethical principles, health professionals sometimes impose their own values on others.

But as Arthur Schafer, a bioethicist from the University of Manitoba, says, "A competent adult is entitled to take some risks with his or her life and even to follow a course of action that may produce serious self-injury." The Jehovah's Witness who refuses a life-saving blood transfusion is a good example of this. A competent adult who knows the potential outcomes of the decision can choose to place one set of beliefs and values above all others, at the risk of serious illness or even death. Although doctors who are trained to do good may not understand this, is it not their responsibility to uphold the patient's right to make such a personal decision? We believe so. Indeed, doctors who take such matters into their own hands in an attempt to "do good" may do their patients harm in some other way. It is their duty to respect your autonomy. We believe that you have the right to make your own decisions about your own health care as long as these decisions do not harm others.

## WHY YOUR RIGHTS ARE SOMETIMES VIOLATED

Although it might seem that your right as a competent adult to make your own decisions about your health care ought to be absolute, there are times when it is difficult for you to exercise it. Some of the reasons are legitimate ones, others less so. And some become more of a problem as you get older.

First, paternalism in medical care can increase dramatically with your advancing age. There is a protective aura that surrounds some of the advice you will receive as an older adult, because health professionals regard you as more vulnerable. The reality is, however, that older people *are* more vulnerable, on average, because of their greater need for health care and because of how old age is viewed in North American society.

Another reason why it may prove difficult to maintain control over your own decisions is that doctors often perceive older people as less competent to make choices. This perception is based on their past involvement with so many people whose mental competence has, indeed, decreased with age. Although at the age of sixty-five, right around most people's retirement, only 5 percent of people suffer from a significant mental impairment, by the time you reach the age of eighty-five, the likelihood of significant impairment has quadrupled. You probably see yourself as being among the unimpaired majority, but doctors tend to see in their practices the people who are the most impaired of all; so doctors may unthinkingly generalize by perceiving all older adults as suffering from deteriorating mental competence. This somewhat frightening attitude is a significant argument in favor of not waiting until you are older to make some of your decisions.

Clearly, whether we like it or not, there is at least a degree of legitimacy in the conclusion that age impairs the ability to make decisions that might affect the person's health or welfare. What needs to be remembered is that every person is an individual, but this concept is sometimes hard for health professionals and families to put into practice.

The third factor that affects your ability to be autonomous is related directly to your deteriorating health as you age. If you are lucky, your health will not deteriorate much and you will not develop chronic conditions that require the services of a variety of medical specialists. But if you are like the majority of aging North Americans, you will be visited by a number of conditions, each of which will be treated by a different specialist. The oncologist who specializes in the care of people with cancer will not treat your arthritis, and the rheumatologist who is treating your arthritis will not adjust your diet to deal with your slight diabetes, and the endocrinologist who is seeing you for your diabetes will certainly not be able to do your surgery should you fall and break a hip, and on and on.

Health care delivery is very fragmented in North America; in other societies you would be seen by fewer, less specialized practitioners. Here your many doctors and their allied health professional assistants have your best interests in mind but they often don't talk to one another on a regular basis. They talk to you, but you can hardly make an adequate health care decision if you have to absorb and analyze all the information that is coming from so many specialists. The result is that you abdicate, at least to some extent, your right to make your own decisions.

What you need is to get your team to talk to one another and have one of them give you advice based on all the treatment regimes. Or get your family doctor involved as your liaison. In a hospital setting the patient advocate can help you to regain some control.

Finally, the factor that is perhaps the most legitimate reason of all for you to give up your right to decide is the need to protect others. Just as the need to protect others must sometimes override an HIV-infected patient's right to privacy, so too can some of the effects of aging call for your autonomy to be set aside.

For example, if you develop Alzheimer's disease, you will not be physically debilitated in the early stage of the disease. The primary symptom will be uncharacteristic memory loss, and you may decide to remain as independent as possible. If you live alone in a detached house, then the only person likely to be harmed if an unattended fat fryer catches fire, for example, is you, provided the fire is contained either by you or by the fire department. But if you live in an apartment building or with others who could also be harmed, your right to choose independence is called into question.

The need to protect others also enters the picture when aging patients neglect to tell their doctors something. This is a particularly difficult situation for a doctor. Patients usually feel revealing this information might result in the doctor recommending something they are not prepared to accept. For example, you might recognize that your eyesight is failing and neglect to mention it to your family doctor or put off going for an eye examination for fear of having your driver's license revoked. If the doctor suspects your eyes need attention, you are not really within your rights to refuse to be tested. Your right to decide for yourself does not include ignoring your failing eyesight until there's an accident. You may have the right to harm yourself, but you certainly do not have the right to harm others.

Although there are many potential obstacles to your rights to self-determination, you still have the right to participate in finding solutions to the conflicts surrounding them. After all, it is you who must live with the outcomes.

It seems, then, that the exercise of your rights is neither simple nor straightforward. Your rights are only available because other people, through society, have granted them to you. In order for something to be your right, there must be some mechanism (as in the case of legal rights) obliging others to allow you to obtain what you have a right to. Other people, however, are not the only ones who have responsibilities; as the holder of a right, you also have some accountability. Everything has a price.

## WITH EVERY RIGHT, A RESPONSIBILITY

People have the right to some basic level of health care, and it is the duty of health professionals to provide you with this service. You have a corresponding duty to take on some responsibilities in your health care. If you are to fully exercise your right to make your own decisions, then you have to do your share. Here are some of those responsibilities.

You have a duty to provide full disclosure of all pertinent information to a health professional with whom you enter into a helping relationship. It is impossible for a practitioner to make an adequate diagnosis of your condition or to advise you appropriately if you have failed to give details of your health that might affect the assessment.

For example, if you complain to your doctor of abdominal pain, your doctor will probably ask you about family history of bowel disease. Do not neglect to tell the doctor that your father and brother both died of cancer of the bowel. This piece of information will make the doctor's job considerably easier and will make the outcome better for you.

You have a duty to comply with the medical treatment plan devised by the health professionals caring for you. If you refuse to follow the advice given to you (which is your right), you may also have to give up other opportunities for care in the future. If you have serious heart disease that is aggravated by your continuing smoking, you give up your opportunity to be considered for a heart transplant under the policies of many transplant programs.

But this issue of non-compliance, as doctors call it, can get a bit more complicated as you get older. There is a difference between willfully disregarding good medical advice and simply being unable to follow it. The implications for the exercise of further rights are obviously different in each case.

Willful disregard, sometimes called non-adherence, is not a result of either failure of the doctor to explain it fully or the individual's inability to understand it. In some cases the patient believes there are simply too many drugs prescribed; in others, the therapy may be painful.

In contrast, some patients fail to follow the medical treatment plan because they cannot. The reasons for being unable to comply may be lack of understanding of the instructions or simply forgetting. Forgetting can be a particular problem for older people and, on its own, it is not within our power to control. But one solution is to enlist the help of family members or friends, for example, to help you remember what to do.

You have a duty to practice good health habits as far as possible. As an informed adult of the late twentieth century, you can hardly claim that you didn't have access to information about how to improve your health by adopting good lifestyle practices. For the past two decades, health promotion and disease prevention information has been readily available all around you, from the brochure racks in front of the dispensary at your local pharmacy to the nightly news broadcasts. If you are going to exercise your right to decide for yourself about how you will be treated, from a medical point of view, you have a responsibility to stay as healthy as possible.

Even if it has not been your habit at younger ages (this is particularly true of men), now is the time to begin regular check-ups for your general health, including eye exams. You need to modify your diet if it is not as healthy as you know it should be. You need to control your weight, give up smoking and consume alcohol in moderation. You need to protect yourself from HIV infection (this is going to be a problem even for older adults as time goes on) and other sexually transmitted diseases. Begin and maintain a habit of regular exercise, and keep your mind as active as possible by staying interested in something. Taking seriously your responsibility for maintaining your health will help you to feel in control.

While it is easy to list off these health practices, you may find it more difficult as you age to follow them on your own. This is an ideal opportunity to get your overly concerned family involved in your welfare in a positive way!

For many medical practitioners who are intimately acquainted with the current ethical dilemmas in health care delivery, the patient's right to decide is far above all others. In practice, however, many doctors find it difficult to balance autonomy against what they believe is best. This is why your decision to refuse treatment, particularly life-sustaining treatment, can be particularly painful for the medical practitioner. Part 4 contains more discussion of this option.

# 5 Other Health Care Rights

THE RIGHT TO DECIDE is only one of the rights you have in regard to health care. We need to examine the other very important rights that you can and most often should choose to exercise.

Consumers' rights groups and patients' rights groups have developed detailed lists of the rights of patients within the health care system. You may wish to contact them and explore their ideas. Here we will examine what we believe are the most basic of your rights as a patient:

- the right to safety;
- the right to privacy;
- the right to be informed as a basis for consent.

## THE RIGHT TO SAFETY

Just as you have a right to safety in other consumer areas such as cars, toys and food, you also have a right to safety in the delivery of your health care. Since most medical approaches have built-in risk factors, this can sometimes be a difficult right to exercise. Most countries have laws that are designed to protect you from quacks, charlatans, incompetent health professionals and money-hungry medical manufacturers. For the most part these laws work, and safety is a given in North American health care delivery. In any case, no one disputes your right to it. You can feel confident in demanding that your every encounter with a doctor, nurse, pharmacist or other health care worker be a safe one.

Nonetheless, in an open society there will always be those who try to get away with fraud, and their favorite victims are the sick and the old. One medical writer describes medical quackery as "the single most harmful crime against the elderly." In 1984, after a four-year study of the problems, a congressional sub-committee in the U.S. called health fraud against the elderly a $10-billion-a-year scandal.

The unpleasant consequences of quackery and fraud may threaten an individual's personal safety, or they may be confined to the pocketbook. The traveling medicine show and snake oil salesman may be things of the past, but their descendants flourish and prey on those who are most vulnerable. Even with laws in place, you must assume some responsibility yourself for protecting your right to safety.

## MEDICAL QUACKERY

As we age, our bodies begin to deteriorate. We look for solutions to our health problems: the fountain of youth, the miracle cure, a comfortable death. Although mainstream medical science has developed to the point where it can help us with many of our maladies, it has fallen short of meeting all of our needs, especially in our later lives. So, it is hardly surprising that many of us look to other sources for help. And the promise of such help does indeed come to us in a variety of guises.

Madeleine F. was sixty-seven years old when her husband died of advanced heart disease. According to her doctor he had suffered from ischemic heart disease, the condition that results from a build-up of fatty material inside the arteries of the heart muscle until blood can no longer circulate and the person has a myocardial infarct, a heart attack. Her husband had suffered two heart attacks, the last one while awaiting bypass graft surgery, and it had been fatal.

About a month after the funeral, Madeleine was reading her mail and discovered a piece that caught her eye immediately because it asked the question: Are you afraid of heart disease? Naturally, she was curious and began reading the enclosed literature. The well-designed brochure described the services of a practitioner in "chelation therapy." She had never heard of this before and wondered why.

The brochure went on to explain that chelation therapy involved the intravenous infusion of a drug called EDTA (ethylene diamine tetraacetic acid) that would dissolve small blockages in the arteries of the heart to prevent further build-up and subsequent heart attacks. Although the therapist was evidently not a doctor, the literature indicated that he was trained in this preventive approach. The cost of the procedure was $4,000.

Madeleine called her insurer to see if it was covered. There were no ifs, ands, or buts about it; it was not an insured service. Her fear of heart disease, however, overtook her fear of the bill. She called the clinic and made an appointment.

Madeleine went to the clinic a month later and spent several comfortable hours being infused with this drug. A day later she was admitted through the emergency room of her local hospital with shortness of breath and chest pain. Three days later she died from a pulmonary embolus; a blood clot that had formed in her vein broke away and lodged in her lung.

Although not all fraudulent medical treatment is fatal, and much of it is actually quite benign, there are significant problems. One investigator of medical fraud defines quackery as "anything that claims too much in the field of health." Another says it is "purposeful misinformation about health and health care products." While some medical quackery and fraud is simply silly and annoying, some of it robs its victims of money, sometimes lots of it, and their health, sometimes even their lives. One of the most frightening problems associated with medical fraud is that the products and their claims can cause people with real medical problems to delay seeking legitimate help until it is too late.

As a group, older adults are much more likely to shop by mail order than any other population group. It is easy, comfortable and fun. Direct marketers know this, and so do people offering quack cures for everything from hair loss to arthritis. As the North American population ages, this method of marketing will become even more popular, making health fraud an increasing problem. At present, about 60 percent of mail fraud victims are over sixty-five, and logic suggests that if we fail to take action, this number will increase. Although the mail is not the only avenue for advertisers of useless medical products, it is becoming increasingly popular.

What kinds of quackery are you most likely to see? Many are drug-related products that promise to either cure or prevent any number of ailments. They may be drugs that are designed to be ingested orally, injected or applied as ointments. Some of these preparations have never been approved for any use by the Food and Drug Administration in the U.S. or the Health Protection Branch in Canada; others have been approved for limited purposes. For example, EDTA, the drug used in Madeleine's chelation therapy, is approved for limited use in removing toxic metals from the bloodstream but not for prevention or treatment of ischemic heart disease. The effectiveness of these preparations may be the first concern to the consumer, but their safety or lack of safety should be an even greater concern. Since the standard required tests have not been done, they lack the safeguards of the mainstream products.

Another large group of useless products consists of nutritional supplements and vitamins. Many of these promise to be a fountain of youth and are often advertised by using fabulous testimonials from satisfied customers. Although many of these nutritional products are not particularly dangerous to most people, they are, at the very least, expensive and ineffective.

Then there are the useless medical devices such as

Oriental sandals, magnets and copper bracelets that purport to cure everything from headaches to arthritis. These are advertised in newspapers, magazines, on television and by direct mailings.

The fact is that, contrary to many people's beliefs, media outlets that advertise these products do not take steps to verify the truth of the advertisements purchased in their publications. The burden is on the advertiser to provide proof of the claims made; the newspaper or magazine carrying the ad simply pockets the advertising fee. This means that the consumer is really alone in determining the legitimacy and safety of the product.

You may wonder about the "satisfied customers" who provide testimonials for the ads. Are these people lying, or do the products actually work? In fact, medical research has shown us that there is generally a 30 percent placebo effect for any given treatment approach that is not otherwise harmful. If a group of people are provided with pills to cure their headaches, and they believe the pills will be more effective than whatever else they have been using, up to 30 percent of them may have actual improvement in their headaches. The pills may contain nothing more than sugar, but the strongly held belief in their effectiveness is enough to get results. But this does not mean that the treatment is an effective painkiller.

If you are suffering from a medical problem for which you have found little help, there is a chance that one of these products will indeed "work" for you because of the placebo effect — assuming it's harmless. But the advertiser's claim is misleading, and the product will be ineffective for the majority. Remember, 70 percent of those who try the product will end up believing that they have been duped.

What can you do to avoid these traps? Here are some suggestions for protecting yourself from medical fraud:

■ Avoid all health-related products that are advertised to you through direct mailing that you did not request.

■ Be wary of suppliers who say they are fighting against the closed minds of the medical establishment.

■ Avoid products being sold after lectures by the inventor. Keep in your mind the image of the traveling snake oil salesman.

■ Be wary of advertisements in magazines that are designed to look like feature articles. These are ads that you are drawn to initially because they appear to be written by an impartial third party, an independent writer. Look closely at the fine print.

■ If you really want to try something, ask your doctor about the product's known safety. If it is a relatively benign product, your doctor will probably tell you that it is unlikely to be effective but that it will not harm you.

■ If you have determined that the product is not harmful, you can afford the cost and you think it just might help, go for it. Maybe it *will* work for you. But don't complain if you later feel you have thrown away your money. It was your decision.

## THE RIGHT TO PRIVACY

*I will not divulge anything that, in connection with
my profession or otherwise, I may see or hear of the
lives of men which should not be revealed, on the belief
that all such things should be kept secret.*

Hippocrates, The Father of Medicine


You have arrived at the hospital to visit a sick
friend. As you are waiting for an elevator, a group of
doctors and nurses are arriving from the cafeteria on
their way back to work. As you all enter the crowded
elevator, you can't help but hear their conversation.

"Are you going to do that bone marrow on Mrs.
Singh?" one of the nurses asks the resident.

"I'm supposed to, but the fourth-year needs the
experience, and when he tried one the other day on
old Mr. Vlasic, the guy just about bled to death."

You are not the only passenger whose eyebrows go
up. At the next floor, the resident and a nurse get out
and a group of doctors on their rounds get in.

"Who's our next patient?" one of the older doctors
says.

"Mrs. Black, the kidney," says one of the younger
doctors, while everyone else rolls their eyes and
moans.

"Do we really have to see her today? She won't do
anything we tell her. Her blood work was so out of
whack when she came in for dialysis last week that
we had to admit her. People like her shouldn't be on
the dialysis program."

You leave the elevator to see your friend Mrs. Black, whose husband died three weeks ago and who hasn't been eating or sleeping well since. She was admitted to hospital to stabilize her kidney failure. You decide not to add to her distress by telling her what you heard, but you are fervently hoping that you never have to be in this hospital yourself.

If you think this sounds like a far-fetched scenario in a modern hospital, think again.

In this age of computerized information systems, the right to privacy is not necessarily one you can claim in every aspect of life. It has, however, been a fundamental expectation in health care for centuries, in spite of the common disregard for it seen every day. The understanding that anything you reveal to health professionals or that health professionals uncover about you in the course of their work is confidential is a basic building block for trust between a caregiver and a patient. If you thought that your doctor would go to a cocktail party on Saturday night and tell someone about your problems, it is likely that you would not reveal anything that you would not want the world to know about. This pretty well limits what you could talk about with your physician! For it is not only details of your sex life that are private, but also the fact that you have hemorrhoids or dry skin or suffer from an emotional problem. All of this is no one's business but your own and your doctor's.

Codes of ethics that help to guide the moral behavior of doctors and other health professionals today all contain some kind of exhortation about patient confidentiality. It has been so since the days of Hippocrates. The International Code of Medical Ethics, published in 1983, says, "A doctor owes to his patient absolute secrecy on all which has been confided in him or which he knows because of confidences entrusted to him." This sentiment is echoed again and again by codes of ethics for various health professionals around the world.

However, it is now widely accepted that there are limits to an individual's right to privacy. Some of these limits are imposed equally on people from every walk of life and in every age group; others are more of a problem for older people. Doctors have reasons for divulging your secrets, and you may not agree with some of these reasons.

## MODERN EROSIONS OF PRIVACY

Modern health care delivery in North America is complex. The simple doctor-patient relationship — based on paternalism and the ability to treat symptoms while rarely providing cures — has changed dramatically since the beginning of this century. Likewise, the simple notion that your privacy is absolute has become increasingly eroded by factors that could never have been foreseen by anyone, except perhaps George Orwell.

One modern contrivance resulting in threats to the privacy of your health information is the computer. Today there are computers in practically every medical office, clinic and hospital, where they are used for everything from diagnosis to patient database management to billing. In spite of their many advantages, they are a modern menace to confidentiality in health care delivery.

Can you answer the following questions:

■ Do you know what your doctor/clinic/hospital uses computers for? Are they for patient charts, or for word processing and appointment scheduling only?

■ Do you know what kind of information about you those computer files hold? Your diagnosis? Your medical/social/personal history? The results of your laboratory tests?

■ Do you know who has access to the computer files?

■ Is that computer on the receptionist's desk connected to any other computers in anyone else's office in another building or in another city?

■ Do you know how much a bystander can see of the computer screen while standing at the receptionist's desk making an appointment?

If you feel your privacy is being compromised unnecessarily, discuss the problem with your doctor or the facility manager. Serious breaches of confidentiality should be reported to the local licensing authority.

The problems associated with computers in health care delivery are beginning to get ahead of the technology. Before we have a chance to ensure the security of one bit of information, the technology changes and we have to scramble to keep ahead and secure the information yet again. But high-technology computer mishaps are not the only invaders of your privacy. Plain old human foul-ups can cause computer-generated medical records to fall off a garbage truck into the street. These factors erode our confidentiality more or less equally regardless of age or infirmity, but others become more serious the older you get.

Some legal requirements may deprive you of privacy. For example, if you are a bus driver and you are developing a cataract in one or both eyes, the health care worker who discovers your condition probably is obliged to report you to motor vehicle authorities, since you could endanger others. Here there is a conflict between your right to privacy and others' right to safety. In some jurisdictions the responsibility of the doctor goes further than a simple moral obligation to protect others, there is also a legal responsibility.

The rights that others have to safety of their person can be considered more important than your right to privacy, but knowing this does not lessen the impact of the violation of your right. You must understand, however, that you too have a moral obligation. If you are having physical problems that could interfere with your ability to do such things as drive a car, fly a plane or work with dangerous equipment or substances, you need to consider the possible harm that you could do to others if you choose to hide this from your doctor. You will not be able to hide it forever, in any case.

The need for your doctor to supply information to your health, life or automobile insurance company can also chip away at your privacy. Although you may not consider it a breach of your privacy for your doctor to write a letter at your request to your own insurance company, the system has built-in problems. Doctors and nurses may recognize the importance of patient privacy, but will the secretary who opens that letter be as careful as your physician? And what do you know about the system that is used for filing and maintaining those records at your insurance company? Is that letter from your doctor ever left on the top of the filing basket without a file folder to cover it? The more people whose hands those reports pass through, the more likely it is that your privacy will somehow be violated. This is especially true if you live in a small community where the people you deal with are likely to know you.

Another problem in maintaining privacy as you age is the increasingly multidisciplinary nature of health care delivery. Every time you add another caregiver to the list of people who have access to your medical records, there is an increasing likelihood that your privacy will be breached.

Have you ever thought about how many people see your records when you are admitted to the hospital? As a hospital day passes, here is a partial list of the people who could be looking at your chart:

■ the nurse who is assigned to care for you on the 7 a.m. to 7 p.m. shift;

■ the nurse who gives you your pills;

■ the nurse who covers during coffee and lunch breaks;

■ the head nurse on the ward;

- the student nurse who is assigned to you tomorrow;
- the nursing instructor who prepares the assignments for the student nurses;
- the dietitian who is adjusting your diet;
- the clinical pharmacist who is reviewing your medication history;
- the occupational therapist who is designing appliances to assist your arthritic hands;
- your family doctor, who visits once a week;
- the rheumatologist who is caring for your arthritis;
- the rheumatologist's senior resident;
- the rheumatologist's intern;
- the X-ray technician who takes the X-rays of your hands.

We're already up to fourteen, and if you have other medical problems being cared for by other doctors, the numbers will keep increasing. And for different conditions there may be physiotherapists, respiratory therapists, clinical nurse specialists, personnel in the operating room and on and on. There is no doubt about it: the idea that your hospital medical record is confidential is purely relative.

In fact, your medical records may eventually be seen by complete strangers without the slightest connection to you or your health team. Researchers performing large-group studies often have access to information from patient charts. The reports from these studies do not identify any particular patients, but the researchers have seen your name and vital information, and they can and do read anything on your chart that catches their fancy. Even if they keep it to themselves, you have not authorized them to see it at all.

This phenomenon is an increasing problem for older patients because scientists need data about aging. As our population ages, more health and social problems loom on the horizon. Medical practitioners and health policy analysts require information about the health needs of the public. As admirable as this is, the safeguards of your privacy may not be a stringent as you would like them to be.

Finally, one of the most common threats to your privacy is painfully close to home. Because of the persistent paternalism of health care workers, it is very common for an older person's spouse or children to be told about results of diagnostic tests, for example, before the patient. If you want to be the first (or the *only* person) to know, you need to make these caregivers aware of your position. Even then, it is possible that a secretary or other person, perhaps believing you are less than capable, may tell your family information that he or she feels they should know. Your family, then, poses special problems for your right to privacy.

## CONFIDENTIALITY AND YOUR FAMILY

There is an increasingly common view in health care that the family rather than the individual person is the patient to be treated. If that view matches your own, all is well. But if it does not, you will be up against a somewhat modified notion of what patient privacy really entails. For all its charms, this notion of family-centered care, embraced by authors of nursing textbooks for two decades, could have its drawbacks for you as a patient.

There may be many advantages to having your family play a part in your health care as you age. But your doctor and your family need to hear clearly from you what role others should play and how much they can be permitted by you to know. If your health deteriorates and new caregivers enter the picture, each of them needs to know your wishes as well. This can be a communication problem of epic proportions that may never be resolved to your satisfaction.

It can be very useful for you to agree to having information about your medical condition shared with specific members of your family as you age but it is *your choice*. There are some specific advantages to having a trusted family member privy to your medical condition and treatment. A relative can:

- help you to evaluate and interpret the doctor's instructions and advice;
- act as an advocate for your wishes and preferences when faced with previously unknown health care workers;
- help you to follow your medication and treatment plan;
- help you to protect you from yourself as your health (including such things as your memory) deteriorates.

But as long as you are in control of your faculties and are competent, you have the right to control this situation and to choose which members of your family will be privy to your medical condition and what information they can and cannot be told directly by your doctor. As you build a relationship with each health professional, your confidence about your having privacy preserved will contribute to the trust that you can place in that caregiver.

## THE RIGHT TO BE INFORMED

All consumers have a right to be informed about the goods and services they use. Health care services are no different. From a medical practitioner's point of view, information forms the basis for "informed consent." In other words, you have the right to give consent to medical procedures but, before you do that, the person asking for that consent has the responsibility to ensure that you know enough about the issues to give that consent. The act of obtaining consent is not the hard part for the doctor. The difficult part from both the doctor's and the patient's perspective is giving and getting all the right information the right way.

George W. is a sixty-two-year-old accountant with a history of heart disease. For the past ten years, he has followed his specialist's advice. He has stopped smoking, he has reduced his workload although he has not yet retired, he has adjusted his diet, and he has taken his pills to reduce his high blood pressure. George has a family history of heart disease and now, despite his attempts to avoid heart surgery, his most recent cardiogram indicates further damage. Alice Chen, his heart specialist, wants to carry out another diagnostic procedure to see how bad the damage is and what they might do to fix it. Dr. Chen, the cardiologist, is sitting behind the desk in her well-appointed office explaining to George what he will be consenting to and what might follow.

"Your ECG indicates a degree of myocardial damage, but we can't determine the extent of potential vessel lesions without a cardiac cath."

"A cardiac cath?" says George in bewilderment. He is still a bit shell-shocked by the news that all his good intentions and lifestyle changes have not had the desired effect on his heart disease; and although he knows he has heard the term "cardiac cath" somewhere before, he can't remember what it means.

"You'll go to the Diagnostic Imaging Department. We'll pass a catheter into your femoral artery and thread it up through your aorta and into the left ventricle of your heart. We'll inject a radiopaque dye through the catheter into the coronary vessels. Then we'll be able to see the blockage on the screen," Dr. Chen forges on.

"There's a risk of interference with the electrical conduction system of your heart and bleeding, but we do hundreds of these every year with very few problems. Then we'll know if you need an angioplasty or a coronary artery bypass graft — but we'll talk about that when we get to that point. Do you have any questions?"

George is so confused and dumbfounded that he doesn't know what to ask first. Knowing that he is a bright, well-educated man, Dr. Chen takes the silence to mean that all is clear. She makes the arrangements and tells George that she'll see him in the Diagnostic Imaging Department at the hospital when the date is confirmed.

It's probably as clear as mud to George. No matter how bright you are, if you're not a cardiologist or perhaps a nurse who specializes in heart disease, you probably would not know what Dr. Chen was talking about, let alone have all your questions answered.

First, she hasn't noticed that George is probably not ready for a discussion of this procedure, as he is still trying to deal with the idea that his heart disease has worsened. Second, her use of medical terminology and jargon does not help one bit in the clarification of meanings. Third, she moves so quickly through the description of the procedure to a cursory and vague mention of associated risks that the patient has little time to assimilate anything. Finally, Dr. Chen doesn't mention what the possible outcomes of the treatment would be, or whether it will make any significant difference to George's life, or if his survival will be longer than if he is treated more conservatively with medication alone. If George doesn't know about possible treatment and results up front, how can he be expected to make decisions about potentially dangerous diagnostic procedures?

## THE DOCTOR'S PROBLEM

Why is it that doctors and many other health professionals have trouble giving information to patients? One of the biggest problems is that, for many years, communication skills were not valued in medical students. Apart from learning how to interview a patient to find out about a medical history and current problems, medical students were trained with a scientific mentality. There is nothing inherently wrong with being scientific — in fact, it helps in analysis and problem-solving — but it doesn't help to develop the "art" of medicine.

So doctors have not been known as great communicators. Although this is changing to some extent in the medical schools of today, most doctors now practicing never had the opportunity to learn effective ways to communicate with patients on a level that those patients can understand. Communicating with their peers may be simple for many doctors, but making that same information understandable to the majority of their patients can be much more difficult.

How do you know that you are getting all the information that you need? In judging an individual encounter with your doctor, try answering these questions:

- Did the doctor listen to you?
- Did the doctor respond to your specific questions or continue on with his or her own agenda?
- Did the doctor use words and ideas that you understand?
- Did the doctor explain any medical terms and jargon he or she may have used?
- Did the doctor go slowly enough through the explanation that you could keep up with it?
- Did the doctor stop during the explanation and invite questions?

- Did the doctor write something down or give you a readable brochure or other printed information so that you could take it home to digest it and discuss it with a family member?

- Did the doctor allow you to explain what you understood so that he or she could correct any misconceptions?

- Did the doctor know about your feelings and any issues that may be important in your life right now?

If, after any given encounter, you answered no to any of these questions, then there is a good probability that you did not get all the information that you need in the way you need it. Tell your doctor or other caregiver that you did not understand and, using these questions as guidelines, suggest what the communication problem might be. You have a right to be fully informed before making a decision, and you should also inform the doctor of any fact that could influence this decision.

## MEDICAL EXPERIMENTATION

The right to informed consent may be lost sight of in the increasingly frequent cases where doctors and patients are "invited" to participate in medical research. If you are asked to consider joining a research study, make sure you get *all* the information you need — including your doctor's motivation.

Malcolm J., sixty-two, has a long history of high blood pressure. His medications are reviewed every year by his family doctor, and his blood pressure has been quite stable for the past couple of years. His main concern about his treatment now is the cost. He worked for many years for a private hardware retailer; now he has a very limited income and is finding the escalating costs of his daily drugs more and more difficult to cope with.

Arriving in his family doctor's office, he notices the new computer equipment and mentions it to his doctor. She explains that it has been installed on the premises so that the doctors in the practice could be part of a drug study. In fact, the study is of a specific drug for high blood pressure, and Malcolm is an ideal candidate. The doctor tells Malcolm that if he agrees to participate in the study, he will receive his drugs free of charge for the next six months. It is a tempting offer. If the medication works, and it probably will, Malcolm's doctor is likely to keep him on the drug at the end of the free trial, and he will discover that new drugs are often even more expensive than the old ones.

For the pharmaceutical company, this is good marketing, as hypertension is a chronic problem involving long-term medical management. The patient will probably be paying for the medication for years. Also, the doctor is only human, and the gift of a new computer may make her feel more favorably disposed to that drug company. This may have effects on her prescribing practices.

This story is a composite of situations that happen all across the continent every week of every year. Because the study in this case is a post-marketing study, Malcolm's drug has already been approved for use by government agencies; it is relatively harmless and in fact useful to him. But not all studies are so benign, and there are some very serious concerns about the ability of a person in this situation to make a good, informed decision about participating.

Knowing when to participate as a subject in a research study and when to refuse can be a dilemma for most people, and more so for the older individual. For physicians, too, the choice may be difficult; they are under increasing pressure from their professional associations to avoid conflicts of interest, but each doctor is an individual and has to evaluate each situation to come to a decision about assisting drug companies in this process.

One factor to be considered is the importance of research involving aging subjects. For many years, medical researchers didn't seem to have much interest in research on older adults, with the exception of studying specific disease processes. Even then, however, that research was far lower in profile than that focusing on breakthroughs in high-technology medicine. In fact, this area of research has been regarded by some as unrewarding and uninteresting. That is beginning to change.

As the population of North America ages, there is more interest in how the human body deals with advancing years and in diseases that are more prevalent in older people. In the past, little attention has been paid to finding out how drugs and treatments might affect aging bodies; most studies have involved male subjects in younger age groups. Medical research in general has begun broadening its base of subjects to consider the differences in both gender and age groups. The increased attention is welcome, but it has brought with it some sources of concern.

Researchers must be wary of the ethical problems of experimenting on older people, and older adults themselves must look out for their own interests. The mind of the die-hard researcher is hell-bent on acquiring subjects. Using older people in institutions is especially convenient, but even those not living in institutions can be vulnerable. This attitude is the crux of the problem for you, the health care consumer, as you try to make a decision about your part in research projects.

Although health professionals base their practice on the principles of respect for human beings and the concepts of doing good and doing no harm, these may not be as clear when the treatment offered is experimental. Most health care facilities have review boards for determining the ethics of research projects. If you are being considered as a subject for a research project in either a hospital or a long-term care facility, you should inquire about the procedures that govern the conduct of such projects. If, however, the project is being conducted out of a private physician's office, you may need to be even more wary.

The main problem that you face is trying to decide if you are able to give truly informed consent without feeling any sense of subtle coercion. *You are not required to take part in these projects if you do not feel comfortable doing so.* You need freely offered information about the objective of the research, the protocol and the potential risks to you during the study and after. You also need to know if being a part of the

82

research is going to interfere with any of your other health care or your own lifestyle.

One of the most difficult parts of this puzzle is that the researcher cannot estimate accurately the level of the risk that you might face. If the risk were absolutely clear, then the treatment would not still be experimental. The only information that could be gleaned from the study would be whether the drug would actually work for you.

Clearly, research needs to be done using older subjects. If we did not research the effects of new drugs on the elderly, then either drug doses meant for younger individuals would be used and might not be safe, or older people might be denied the possible benefits of newer drugs. You need to weigh the risks to you as you understand them against the possible benefits either to you or to others. Even if you do not benefit at the present time, the research might result in benefits in the future for your children or others. You simply need to feel comfortable about what you are getting yourself into.

Here are some questions you should be able to answer:

- Has the purpose of the study been explained to you?

- Has your involvement been clearly outlined? Do you know what treatment you will receive? Do you know what tests you will have to undergo? Do you know how many times you will need to be seen in follow-up?

- Has any potential risk to you been clearly outlined?

- Do you understand all of the above explanations?
- Have you discussed your participation with a trusted family member?
- Is the risk acceptable to you?
- Do you understand the potential benefits of the study to you or others?
- Do you feel comfortable that you are making a free choice in agreeing to participate?

If you answer yes to all the above questions, then you may be able to consent to participating in a study and feel good about that decision. If you answer no to any of them, you should seriously question your ability to make an informed decision about giving your consent. If the whole affair is simply causing you anxiety, you probably don't need the aggravation: say no.

# 6 : Planning Ahead

**N**OW THAT YOU UNDERSTAND your rights, start exercising them in a useful way. Make some plans that will protect your rights in future years.

Gloria J. is fifty-two years old. With the exception of a few years before she was married, when she was a teacher, she has devoted her life to her three daughters and her husband, a dentist, who is turning sixty this year. She has just read a newspaper article about a family who have asked the doctors to remove their mother from a ventilator that is breathing for her and, in their words, "is prolonging her death, not her life."

It seems to Gloria that if she has a right to make decisions that will affect her life and health, then she also has a right to make decisions about her potential illness and eventual death. She knows, for instance, that she would not like to be kept alive on a machine. She decides to broach the subject with her husband, who says he's with her whatever decisions she makes. But her daughters, who are more likely to be the ones left behind, are less supportive. Their beliefs in modern medical technology and the relative unreality of mortality seem to be clouding their ability to see things through their mother's eyes.

Gloria doesn't know what to do. One day, while at her doctor's office for a routine physical exam, she notices a brochure on the rack. It is about the "living will," a document that indicates what kind of health care you wish, and referred to more frequently as an advance directive. Gloria has never heard the term before and it interests her immediately. By the time her doctor is ready for her, she knows that she does have the right to make her own decisions before she is incapable of making them, and she decides to enlist both her doctor's and her lawyer's help in ensuring that her daughters do as she wishes.

Gloria is well ahead of many of us. We refuse to think about the possibility that there may come a time when we are no longer capable, as a result of either mental or physical incapacity, of making our own decisions. It's a little like feeling that you're not going to die, at least for a very long time, and thus neglecting to purchase life insurance. It's only when it's too late that we or, more likely, our families realize that we should have done something sooner. When you neglect to make health care decisions before the fact, you jeopardize your quality of life, your health, your right to a dignified death (if any death can be considered dignified) and your right to decide for yourself. Clearly, there's a lot at stake.

Advances in medical technology over the past two or three decades have made these decisions even more crucial today, and they will continue to become more complex. This technology allows doctors to keep you "alive" much longer and in much more serious conditions than they ever could previously. When, as a result of your condition, you can no longer play an active role in the decision to treat or not to treat you with these marvels, you need to be certain that your thoughts and wishes are followed to the extent possible.

## THE BEST TIME TO DECIDE

Without a doubt, the best time to make some general decisions about your own health care is now, while you are still competent enough to read this book and can clearly and rationally look at how you would like to be treated when you can no longer have an active voice in your health care. If you fail to think about it, you will have left your family in an uncomfortable dilemma. Then it will be difficult for them to figure out if they are making decisions in your best interests or in their own. More important, however, is that the medical personnel cannot determine in whose interests they are making these decisions if they have no evidence of what you would have wanted.

If you are in an accident, for example, and sustain a severe head injury, you may be in a coma and on an artificial ventilator. If your relatives wonder whether the ventilator should be discontinued, they face a whole series of dilemmas, from deciding if they could afford your care if you remain alive but completely non-responsive, to deciding upon the morality of prolonging your inevitable death while depriving you of any quality of life. Without some prior indication

87

from you of your wishes, they have little to go on but their own thoughts and feelings, which are likely to have significant emotional overtones.

Researchers in Boston asked two groups of people how they felt about preparing an "advance directive" about their health care. In other words, how did they feel about preparing a legal document that would set out directions for health care workers in the event that they were unable to do so? One of the groups consisted of hospital outpatients and the other, members of the general public.

Although many people believe that only older people are interested in thinking about these kinds of decisions, the study showed just the opposite. About 90 percent of both groups said they would like to have this kind of document. Those who were young and healthy were at least as likely as those over sixty-five and in poorer general health to wish to prepare advance directives. Another interesting finding of that study is the reason most often given for not preparing such a document: people said that their family doctors had never mentioned the possibility. Doctors are far more interested in your medical history, it seems, than in your medical future. Thinking ahead has evolved into a patient responsibility.

It's unclear how many people have already signed advance directives. In 1988 an American Medical Association survey found that 15 percent of the people responding had actually written a living will; 56 percent had at least told their families their wishes in the event of terminal illness or irreversible coma.

These figures showed a significant increase over the results of a poll taken seven years earlier.

It's never too early to think about your wishes. Certainly this isn't a discussion topic only for the very old and ill. You are probably in the best position you will ever be to gather the information necessary to make good decisions, before health problems overwhelm you. If you wait too long, you will be leaving a great deal up to chance.

## WHAT TO DECIDE ABOUT NOW

Obviously, you cannot be prepared for every specific eventuality. Even if a crystal ball *could* tell you exactly what fate has in store for you, would you really want to know?

This chapter lists some of the issues that can be thought out and decided upon today, both general decisions and decisions about ten specific medical procedures that you may or may not wish to undergo. These decisions can form the basis for developing an advance directive.

## PREPARING AN ADVANCE DIRECTIVE

### General Decisions

- How much should your family be involved?

- What type of long-term care would you prefer?

- Where would you prefer to spend your final days of life?

- Would you be willing to donate organs and tissues?

## Specific Medical Procedures

Under what circumstances would you want:

- Pain control/palliative care
- Hospitalization
- Intravenous fluids
- Diagnostic tests
- Antibiotic therapy
- Surgery
- Breathing machines (artificial ventilators)
- Intensive care
- Resuscitation (CPR)
- Tube feeding

You may find this exercise difficult, even depressing; but keep in mind that if these were happy decisions that you had to make, you probably would need little help making them. The benefits of making some of these decisions now can be peace of mind for you and an easier time for your family when you can no longer help them.

## GENERAL DECISIONS

Start by considering these quite broad questions.

**Family Involvement:** To what extent do you wish your family to be involved in your decisions if you become unable to make them later on?

When Gloria began to do some thinking about her own advance directive, she knew that she didn't want her daughters to feel that she didn't trust them to make good decisions. On the other hand, she wasn't at all certain that she would be able to convince them about her general attitudes. The idea of leaving the decisions entirely up to them made her feel uncomfortable, and so she decided that she would be explicit in her statement that her written provisions should prevail over her daughters' wishes.

**Long-term Care:** In general, how do you feel about nursing homes? Under what circumstances would you want to be cared for in a nursing home? Consider your overall feelings about nursing homes as well as financial and geographic concerns.

Gloria had seen her mother in a nursing home. Although her mother had been generally well cared for in her final days, Gloria wasn't certain she wanted to live in one herself. With a secure financial situation, she preferred private, in-home care. She decided to include in her document provisions about how long that kind of care could go on before she believed she could be moved to an extended-care facility. (See chapters 8 and 9 for more on long-term care.)

**Final Days:** Would you rather die in a hospital or in your own home? This may or may not be within your control, but you can make your preference clear.

Gloria thought that she would rather die in her own home, but she didn't think that her daughters could cope with it. This time, she decided to make things easier for them; she stated that her preference was to die in hospital if at all possible.

**Organ and Tissue Donation:** If the possibility exists, would you like to donate organs or tissues for transplantation to others? The need for organs and tissues currently far outdistances their availability, and the gap is certain to grow wider as time goes on. In many jurisdictions, laws dictate that medical personnel must ask families for permission to remove usable organs and tissues. This is not a decision to be left to overwrought relatives.

In any event, your age at death and the cause of your death may result in none of your organs or tissues being usable anyway. Organ donors (primarily those who donate hearts, kidneys, livers and lungs) must die in a hospital of a brain injury; they must be in good general health and free of any infection. Some transplant centers will not use organs or tissues of people who have had cancer. Most organ donors are between eighteen and thirty-five and die in motor vehicle accidents. It is possible, however, for donors to be much older and to die of such conditions as blood clots in the brain. Tissues (corneas, bone, skin) are not subject to the same restrictions, and it is quite conceivable that older adults could donate them.

You can make your wishes known about donation by signing an organ/tissue donor card, which is part of your driver's license in many states and provinces. But it will be helpful all around for you to include a statement on the issue in your advance directive as well.

## SPECIFIC MEDICAL PROCEDURES

Deciding what procedures you do or do not want as you near the end of your life is not a simple matter of looking at a list and saying yes to some and no to others. You may feel differently about any of them depending upon what your condition is at the time.

There are three medical scenarios in which you would be incapable of making a decision or expressing your wishes about specific medical procedures. First, you may find yourself without warning in a critical, life-threatening condition, but not necessarily a terminal one. For example, you have a heart attack while driving your car and are taken to the emergency department, where you arrive unconscious. Decisions about how to treat you and the extent of that treatment have to be made on short notice by medical personnel who probably do not know you, together with your family.

If such a situation befalls you, your attitudes may be influenced by your age. At fifty, you may be more inclined to want aggressive treatment. At seventy-five, you may well believe that dying a sudden, painless death is preferable to being kept alive to die of a painful, chronic illness.

In a second medical scenario, your illness is known to be terminal. There is nothing more medical science has to offer you, and you know you are likely to die of this illness — most frequently, cancer. The exact timing, however, is almost always medically imprecise. Another area of medical imprecision is the inability to predict accurately how you will react to treatments, many of which are almost as unpleasant as the disease itself. Unlike the first scenario, which requires quick action, the chronic illness will probably give you some time to deliberate over specific procedures before you become so debilitated that you cannot make decisions.

The third medical scenario is a very complex one: the irreversible coma. The doctors know that the likelihood that you will recover or even regain consciousness is nil, so you cannot be expected to continue to "live" life as most of us know it. Legally, however, death has not occurred. (For more on definitions of death, see chapter 10.) In an irreversible coma you are unresponsive, but you have some degree of brain activity and may even be able to breathe independently.

The ten specific medical procedures listed below could be used in any or all of the above scenarios. As you consider them, try to judge how you feel about each in the context of each medical scenario. This will help you to make your advance directive as specific as possible.

**Pain Control/Palliative Care:** Under what circumstances would palliative care, including simple pain control, be your choice of treatment? Palliative care is based on the concept that when the disease cannot be treated and thus "cured," the best approach is to treat the person, so that dignity and self-respect are maintained. This approach to care is an orientation that provides medical and nursing personnel with specific guidelines to make you comfortable and to take no extraordinary measures to prolong your life.

**Hospitalization:** Under what circumstances would you agree to be hospitalized? To look at it another way, when would you prefer to be treated at home? A decision on this subject may involve not only you, but your family as well. They might need to be intimately involved with your care if you cannot manage alone. In addition, your financial resources will have to be considered. If your preference is for home care, you may want to factor this into your long-term financial planning.

**Intravenous Fluids:** If your condition deteriorates to the point where you can no longer take food or fluids orally, do you wish to be fed intravenously? Under most circumstances, this will involve primarily fluids; providing total nutrition intravenously is an even more complicated procedure.

If you are dying, providing you with intravenous fluids will simply prolong your dying. Most people who are unconscious and are no longer able to take food or fluids will die not of starvation, as is widely believed, but as a result of dehydration. On the other hand, the use of intravenous fluids generally makes a conscious patient more comfortable.

**Diagnostic Tests:** At what point do you consider it to be futile to subject yourself to any more diagnostic tests? This decision may be easier to make once you have decided whether you want medical treatment at all. If you have decided that you wish only palliative care, it is a waste of time, money and resources to undergo tests to discover problems that you do not wish fixed anyway. As for the tests themselves, some diagnostic tests are non-invasive, but many, including routine blood tests, are both invasive and uncomfortable.

**Antibiotic Therapy:** If you develop an infection (which is likely to hasten your death), do you wish treatment with antibiotics, or would you prefer to be left alone? Antibiotics will prolong your life, or your dying, depending upon your point of view. Depending upon the type of illness that you have and the extent and type of the infection, antibiotics might make you more comfortable, but this is not always so; an advance decision will not cover every specific situation. In the case of an overwhelming infection such as septicemia (generalized blood infection), the resulting death is likely to be swift and painless, and probably preferable to a prolonged, painful illness.

**Surgery:** Would you agree to having surgery? Your answer to this question will certainly vary with the situation. If, for example, you are unconscious and in critical condition, you may wish to have surgery to alleviate the immediate problem, such as an internal injury from an accident. On the other hand, if you are suffering from terminal cancer, you may be less inclined to think that you should have surgery.

Your age and general health may affect your thinking. If you are in critical but not terminal condition at age eighty-five, and suffering severely every day from arthritic pain, you may not be so quick to agree to surgery to save your life. Obviously, this is not a decision you can make once and forget. You should review this part of your directive and adjust your decision based on current conditions.

**Breathing Machines:** How do you feel about being on an artificial ventilator with a tube down your throat and a machine breathing for you? Perhaps your views will be influenced by the medical scenarios; or you may know that this is not how you would like to spend any length of time, regardless of your medical condition.

**Intensive Care:** Would you agree to intensive care treatment? Often, the older you are, the lower down the priority list you are when awaiting ICU beds anyway. Your age and general condition may, again, affect your decision here.

**Resuscitation:** If your heart stops, do you want the nursing and medical personnel to attempt to revive you? This is a very important decision to make, especially if you are a patient in a hospital. When your heart stops at home, we call it a death. When your heart stops in a hospital, we call it a cardiac arrest; and unless someone tells them differently, the team will spring into action and begin cardiopulmonary resuscitation (CPR). Of course there is no guarantee that they will be successful or that you will not be worse off afterwards. For more about "do not resuscitate" orders, see chapter 10.

**Tube Feeding:** How do you feel about being fed by a tube into your stomach? This is particularly likely to become an issue if you are in an irreversible coma. There is really no other way to maintain your nutrition over the long term; tube feeding therefore prolongs your life. Even health professionals have differing opinions about whether tube feeding constitutes medical care or simply personal comfort measures. What do you think?

The first time you make these decisions will no doubt be the hardest, but it should not be the last. Although some people's attitudes do not change, even if they first think about these issues at a relatively young age, you may find that, as you age, you do think about them differently. This is to be expected and welcomed.

The changes in your thinking may reflect new developments in medicine, what has happened to friends or relatives, the changing structure of your family, your beliefs about the allocation of scarce medical resources or your own changing health care needs. Whatever the reason you change your mind, make sure that any document you produce stating your wishes changes along with you. Nothing that you put in writing is carved in stone. Be sure to review it regularly.

## FORMALIZING YOUR DECISIONS

From your point of view, the success or failure of your ability to control your own health care in advance rests on how well you communicate your wishes to those who will be carrying out your requests. One of the first things you should consider is formalizing your decisions.

Now that the idea of finding out how patients want to be treated is being taken more seriously by health care workers, many hospitals in the U.S. and some in Canada have begun asking patients some questions on admission. These responses provide a sort of living will or advance directive, but it can be a bit offputting to be faced with questions about your possible death when you are being admitted to deal only with a minor problem.

Making a formal, written directive in advance of when it must be used in your health care is really the only way we have at present to be somewhat certain that our wishes will be followed when we are not competent to make our own decisions. Advance directives of various kinds have gained increasing acceptance since California became the first state to recognize the concept under its Natural Death Act in 1976.

There are two kinds of advance directives. The first is the living will, a written document that specifies the details of what medical treatment you do or do not want in the scenarios we have outlined. Although there has been some legal (and medical) argument about the extent to which living wills are binding, there is little debate about the fact that you do have both a legal and a moral right to refuse any treatment that you do not want. Even if your state or province does not have specific legislation yet to enforce the legality of your decisions, the fact that you have put your wishes in writing provides medical personnel with moral guidelines, at the very least, about how to treat you.

The durable or enduring power of attorney is the

second way that you can prepare an advance directive. The legal term "power of attorney" means a grant you make to authorize someone to make decisions and act on your behalf; this person is called your proxy. If, for example, you head south every winter for four or five months, you may decide to give your daughter your power of attorney and authorize her to pay your bills from your bank account while you are gone.

The "durable" or "enduring" power of attorney remains in effect after you have become incompetent, authorizing the person you have designated to make, in this case, health care decisions for you. This power differs from the ordinary power of attorney in that the person so designated does not have power to make decisions for you *until* you have become incompetent.

This proxy should, of course, be someone you know well and trust implicitly. Further, a proxy should be someone who you believe understands your perspective and why you have made your decisions. In this case, your proxy will have a much easier time making your decisions when the time comes.

The person to whom you give the durable power of attorney need not be a relative and should not be in a conflict of interest, as perceived by the medical personnel. For example, if the person you designate stands to inherit a large sum of money from you when you die, the doctors and nurses may have a hard time believing that all his or her decisions reflect what you want.

You can strengthen your living will by specifying a proxy with enduring power of attorney. When this person knows your wishes and supports your right to maintain control, you can be more confident that your wishes will be respected.

Start formalizing your decisions by finding out what the laws are in your state or province regarding the actual form of the living will and of the power of attorney. To formalize the durable power of attorney, you need to see a lawyer. This may not be necessary with a simple living will; kits are available in most bookstores to help you to produce such a document yourself.

When you have made your decisions about your health care and explored the legalities, discuss these decisions with your family and your family doctor. When you have completed the paperwork, ask your doctor to place a copy of your living will in your medical record, give a second copy to the person you have designated to make decisions for you, and keep a copy in your own records. Don't bother placing a copy in your safety deposit box, as it would be relatively inaccessible when it is needed.

As mentioned earlier, you should review your directive on a regular basis to keep it up to date. Continue to discuss your decisions with your family whenever you do this review. This ensures that if the document is ever used as the basis for your medical decisions, the health care workers can be reasonably certain that the document reflects your most recent views.

## ENLISTING THE SUPPORT OF OTHERS

One of the reasons many people develop advance directives is that they do not trust their doctors.

Many fear that they will be over-treated against their wishes. Much of this sentiment arises from a general distrust of the large bureaucracy that is our health care delivery system today and the scientific nature of medicine. But your doctor could be a source of information and support for you if you explore these topics with him or her now, before the need arises. You will need both your doctor and your family on your side if you are to be sure that your decisions will actually govern your medical treatment.

Here is a process that may help you to enlist the support that you will need.

Before you start to approach others, make sure you have clear ideas about the decisions you are making and your reasons for making them. Be honest with yourself about why your beliefs and attitudes have evolved to where they are, and never feel that you need to apologize for how you feel about your own health care. You have a right to decide what is right for you, especially when it comes to your health care.

Now explore your family's thoughts and feelings in an informal way. Start with discussions about health care issues in the public eye, especially media stories that raise questions about the decisions you would like to include in your advance directive. Try to get a general idea of how other members of your family feel; don't focus the discussion on your own future at this point. And don't assume that just because you grew up with a sibling or have been married to the same person for thirty years, your values about health and illness care are the same. You may be quite shocked about what you find out.

While you are feeling out your family, open some of the same discussions with your family doctor. Don't be surprised if he or she isn't as receptive to the idea as you might wish. Some doctors are still quite skeptical about the whole notion of advance directives, for a variety of reasons.

Although they may tell you that you have the right to make your own decisions about your health care, some doctors recognize that one of the reasons you feel you need a directive is that you do not trust the health care system and perhaps even your own doctor. Another reason some doctors do not seem supportive of living wills is that many continue to believe that you probably don't know enough to be making these kind of decisions. Certainly you don't know from experience what it is like to be at the end of your life, but then neither does your doctor, at least not as a patient.

Skepticism aside, doctors can be very valuable allies for you in your search for the peace of mind that comes from knowing that your own decisions will be honored. Find out how your doctor feels about advance decisions and then begin to discuss your own particular point of view. If he or she is fairly certain that this is not a temporary whim of yours, your doctor will probably prove a more than willing ally.

Once you have clarified your own attitudes and beliefs, your family's and your doctor's, present your well-thought-out position to your family. Put some of this in writing before beginning the discussion so that they see that you are serious. Keep the communication going and continue to do so even after the legal paperwork is completed.

The final step is extremely important: reinforce the resolve of your allies over the years. Don't be lulled into complacency; continue from time to time to determine if your allies are still with you. Perhaps you will not change any of your ideas or wishes, but something may happen to change the attitude of a family member.

In a study done at the University of Toronto in 1991, 90 percent of hospital outpatients surveyed about advance directives wanted their wishes to be known. You may share with these people their main purpose: you may also fear excessive treatment. In a 1986 study of the same topic, researchers found that proxies were sorely inaccurate when trying to guess the wishes of another person without a previous discussion, and doctors were even worse. It seems, then, that your fears have some justification. The same 1986 study, however, also found that only 6 percent of those surveyed had ever initiated discussions about their wishes with their doctors. Perhaps it is time patients took matters of their own health into their own hands. You're doing it for yourself.

# PART THREE

# Deciding for Others

# 7 : In Their
Best
Interests

**A**S YOU GET OLDER and your family
ages along with you, you may find yourself in the
uncomfortable position of having to make some
health care decisions not for yourself but for someone
else who is no longer capable of doing it — perhaps a
parent affected by aging, or a sibling suddenly struck
by accident or catastrophic illness.

Although you might think at first that it should be
even easier to make decisions for another person
whom you know well, there are many factors that
affect what we do under these circumstances and
why we do them. It isn't simple at all. It is a different
situation altogether to actually see a close relative
who has been deemed incompetent than it is to think
about some future time when you yourself may not
be able to make decisions. In spite of the closeness
you may have always felt and continue to feel with
the other person, there will always be a gap — a
sense of something unknown or missed. Perhaps,
however, you will be able to apply to your own decisions and planning some of the wisdom you gain by
helping others.

## WHEN YOU WILL DECIDE FOR OTHERS

Here are some scenarios that might require you to make a decision for someone else.

- Your fifty-nine-year-old husband has just had a massive heart attack. After rushing him by ambulance to the emergency department, you are confronted by the heart surgeon who has been called in to consult. He tells you that your husband needs an immediate coronary artery bypass graft. Your usually competent husband is unconscious.

- Your seventy-year-old mother has had Alzheimer's disease for several years; recently her condition has deteriorated significantly. She now needs constant nursing supervision, and you know you are not capable of doing it all for her. She can no longer make her own decisions and you need to decide what to do.

- Your sixty-eight-year-old father has bowel cancer, which has spread to his lungs and his brain. His condition has been fairly good up until now, but he has just been admitted to hospital with pneumonia, which the medical staff are treating. The attending physician and the nurses want to know if you wish them to write a "do not resuscitate" order on your father's chart.

- Your sixty-year-old sister has suffered a massive bleed into her brain. She is in intensive care on a ventilator and the neurologist has declared her "brain-dead". A doctor from the transplant program is waving a consent form at you and wishes you to consent to donation of her organs for transplantation. You are her only relative. He says time is of the essence.

Clearly, in some of these situations, the person cannot make a decision for himself or herself. When someone is unconscious, in a coma or brain-dead, there is little argument about that. In other situations, the evidence is not quite so clear. Factors such as the extent of the person's inability to make decisions, the type of medical situation and how well you know the person all play a part in the complexity of making decisions for others.

## WHY IS IT SO DIFFICULT?

There are several important reasons why we are often reluctant to make decisions for others when it comes to health care. First, we treasure personal autonomy, the right to decide for oneself, and it is hard to see it apparently taken away. But something cannot be a right if the individual supposedly holding that right hasn't the capacity to exercise it. For example, it is ludicrous to say that a year-old child has the right to decide whether to be treated for an ear infection, as the child clearly does not have the capacity to decide. The child does, however, have a right to be treated. Someone else, in this case the parents, has the responsibility to see that treatment is provided.

When people cannot make decisions about their own health care any more, they still have the right to be treated, and you may be the one who has the responsibility to ensure that they receive the treatment that they would want. For everyone who has a right, someone else has a responsibility to uphold that right. Simply realizing, however, that you are not really stripping someone of his or her rights doesn't seem to make you feel much better about making those decisions.

Perhaps one of the most important reasons we often feel uncomfortable in these situations is that they awaken in us our own fears about our mortality. As you face disability and death in someone who is close to you, you face it in yourself to some extent. For example, as you look into the eyes of your father, whom you love and looked up to for so many years, and you find yourself having to make decisions for him as he once did for you, you often begin to sense a personal vulnerability. If it can happen to him, it can certainly happen to me, you think.

Another factor that contributes to our discomfort is guilt. We often allow ourselves to feel guilty when we make decisions for others. If, for example, you decide that your mother would be better cared for in a nursing home, you may begin to feel guilty that you are somehow abandoning her. Although she may never have said anything about this and, in fact, may not feel abandoned at all, you still feel guilty.

Well-meaning or personally biased health care workers may ask questions or make statements that will kindle even the smallest bit of smoldering guilt. A doctor who believes in the absolute sanctity of life may ask you if you are unequivocally certain that your father did not change his mind about a living will that he wrote two years ago, indicating the limits he wished placed on his treatment. The doctor may be making a misguided attempt to override the document in order to treat your father, simply because your father's values do not seem in sync with his or her own. Some doctors do not accept the validity of living wills at all. When a person suggests that you "should" do something and you are wondering if that person may be right, ask yourself whether that "should" is really coming from inside you or whether it comes from that outside source. If it is not your doubt, don't accept it.

We may hesitate in these situations because we feel we are, at least subconsciously, acting out of selfishness. It is the desire to avoid being selfish that sometimes makes these decisions difficult. We feel selfish even thinking thoughts such as "Mother has become a burden to the family." It seems inappropriate to admit that the costs for continuing long-term care are astronomical, or that the money that would otherwise be left to you will be eaten up by the nursing home. The fact that these attitudes become obstacles to objective decision-making makes us uncomfortable.

Finally, we often feel that we are taking away some of the other person's human dignity. This dignity is at least partly related to the notion of one's autonomy, which we have already mentioned. It is also related to the fact that illness and the medical care that follows often, in themselves, strip the individual of dignity. We have all had occasion to joke about bedpans and open-backed johnny shirts, but what could be more undignified than seeing those images become real for your mother, father or husband in a time of illness? As if it isn't demeaning enough to be in the relatively powerless position of the patient, it seems to add insult to injury to have to make decisions for another as if he or she were a child.

Making decisions for others is never easy. But most of the reasons are related not to that other person but to ourselves. If we are armed with enough knowledge, that knowledge can help us through a difficult situation. What we need to know about is not only what the person would want, but also what decisions are likely to be required.

## WHAT IS INCOMPETENCE?

When Judith H., sixty-two, made that fateful appointment to see her family doctor about her memory loss, she was frightened that it might lead to a diagnosis that she did not want to hear. Her mother had died from what is now known as Alzheimer's disease, and she had been horrified at the deterioration about which nothing could be done.

Her worst fears were justified. After several months of testing and ruling out all other causes of this uncharacteristic memory loss, her doctor told her that she had early Alzheimer's disease. At that point, Judith was still quite capable of making her own decisions about her medical treatment. She understood the consequences of her actions and, even if others disagreed with her, she still had the right to make decisions.

As time went on, Judith's mental condition did,

indeed, deteriorate. It was a very gradual loss of mental abilities. First she simply forgot things and had to search for words and phrases to say what she meant. Then she became increasingly confused, often forgetting where she was and even the month or the year. Then she forgot how to do common things, like brushing her teeth and dressing herself. Somewhere along the line, Judith lost the ability to make competent, responsible decisions. Neither she nor her family nor her doctor would be able to pinpoint that moment with any degree of accuracy. There is a fine line between competence and incompetence with dementias of aging.

From a medical point of view, then, the loss of competence to make health care decisions is not an absolute. A person may actually be incompetent one day and regain competence the next, depending upon the cause of the problem. The law, however, sees the situation differently. In law, a person is considered to be competent until proven otherwise. The test is similar to the concept of innocent until proven guilty: the burden of proof lies not with those who believe the individual to be competent but with those who believe the individual to be incompetent. The laws in North America seem to provide only general guidelines, and each situation is viewed in relation to its unique circumstances.

A declaration of incompetence is not to be taken lightly. The consequences can be far-reaching and go beyond decisions about health care. In some jurisdictions, for example, a person declared incompetent is no longer allowed to drive a car, vote or manage his or her finances. It is clearly a drastic step and needs serious, rational consideration.

If Judith's family believes that she is no longer able to make responsible decisions about her own health care and she is still in a position to disagree, it is the family's responsibility to take legal action to be able to make decisions in her best interests. But trying to do what is best for another person is always fraught with hazards.

## THE FAMILY'S ROLE

Every family has its own peculiar dynamics, which will affect the role each member plays when someone needs help. Unless you make your family's relationships clear to medical personnel, they have no way of knowing that some members of the family are more equal than others.

For example, Judith's oldest daughter lives nearby and has become a drop-in caregiver. She may decide that Judith needs to be in a nursing home. What are the staff at that nursing home going to do when Judith's youngest daughter, who has lived a thousand miles away for the past ten years, arrives on the scene and demands changes in her mother's care? This daughter has not played an active part in Judith's life in recent years and thus her rights may be different. Judith, however, as the mother of both women, may not see it that way. She may view both her daughters in the same light.

A usurper may gain power with medical and health care personnel simply by threatening a lawsuit or by being particularly difficult to deal with. It is up to Judith's family to straighten out this situation as soon as possible. It's not fair or helpful to leave it up to the nursing home staff, as they may not even realize a family fight could be brewing.

One thing that health professionals keep in mind in these situations is that there is always the potential for conflict of interest between family members and the person who is sick. What might be in the best interests of the individual may not be in the best interests of the family. This is a very important consideration today because, more and more, health professionals are recognizing that the needs and rights of other people may be even more compelling than those of the patient being treated. There is some movement away from the old standard of patient-centered medical ethics to one of societal interest. The most high-profile example of this kind of conflict of interest is the one caused by AIDS. If a husband is HIV-positive and refuses to tell his wife, his right to privacy may not be considered as important as his wife's right to know, so that she can protect herself and any children they might conceive.

In the same way, when an aging person cannot make decisions, the rights of others may have to take precedence over his or her rights. The financial burden on family members of a decision to give costly long-term care, for instance, must be considered. Some, but not all, medical personnel today even consider the patient's family to be an extension of the individual patient. In this way, the family's needs are considered. You need to find out how the health care workers you are dealing with feel about these sorts of issues.

Although the family is intimately involved in the decision-making process for an incompetent person, there are limits to their authority. Those limits may be legal if proxies and powers of attorney are involved, or they may be moral and thus less clear. The patient's doctor has a very important role to play when deciding where the family's authority ends; you and the doctor may not always agree.

Not all family involvement in care need be so problematic. The family can make many positive contributions. For one thing, families have mutual interests. These interests range from esoteric ones such as shared memories and love to more concrete ones such as the house, the car and the family dog. What happens to one person in the family affects all the other members in some way. The fabric of most families is interwoven.

Family members generally have a deep, personal knowledge of one another, unlike that usually shared by non-relatives. Of course, different families have different relationships, but often, even when family members are not what they would call close, they will admit to knowing a great deal about one another. This kind of knowledge is very useful to medical personnel when faced with an incompetent individual.

As mentioned in chapter 3, families often play a very positive role in health care. When you admonish your husband to go easy on the salt at the dinner table, you are playing a role in the control of his high blood pressure (even if he just calls it nagging!). You can play a positive role in overall decision-making for him and for other family members too.

## THE ROLE OF A PATIENT ADVOCATE

An advocate is a person who pleads the cause of another, a kind of middleman. In health care, the concept of the patient advocate — either informally or as a formal job description in hospitals — is gaining in popularity, as people become more and more concerned about their rights within the system. With an incompetent individual for whom others have to make decisions, an objective third party can be enormously useful, especially when there is the potential for a conflict of interest between the family and the patient.

This advocate can be a trusted family friend who is not prejudiced on one side or another. It can be a hospital social worker or a clergy person. It probably isn't a good idea to ask your lawyer to be the advocate in these situations, as the involvement of a legal professional can alienate or threaten the medical staff. The advocate should be someone that you can trust and who knows, at least to some extent, the right questions to ask the medical personnel. This person's job is to interpret the answers to those questions to the family in an objective manner.

Here are some questions the advocate might help to seek answers for:

- What is the patient's prognosis — how long may the person have to live with his or her current medical problems?

- What quality of life might the patient have under the various options being considered?

- What differences of opinion are there among the medical and nursing staff? Different people will see things from their own perspectives, none of which is actually wrong.

Impartiality is very difficult to maintain if the issues are life and death and the decisions are about someone you love. Enlisting a third party can help you to get information and interpret it; and it allows you to vent your feelings and explore your own attitudes and motivations with someone who has no vested interest in the outcome.

## DOING THE "RIGHT" THING

It seems hard enough to do the right thing when the decisions are for ourselves. It is even more difficult to be sure we're right when we are making decisions for others; and when the decisions involve life, health and even death, their importance is multiplied.

As human beings, we have a duty to protect those who cannot protect themselves. It is our belief in this duty that makes us send help to starving children in other countries. It is also this belief that makes us realize that we have not only a legal obligation in some instances, but also a moral obligation to ensure that those who are close to us are cared for in their best interests.

# 8 : Nursing Homes

YOU WALK THROUGH the front door and are immediately assaulted by the smell of disinfectant. As you venture farther inside, you find the sights, sounds and smells even less appealing. The faint odor of urine wafts through an open door. Inside, a pitiful old woman looks up at you and then turns away to gaze down again at her laced fingers. A few others shuffle along the corridor, holding onto the side rails for support. You finally reach a nursing station where white-uniformed figures efficiently pour pills and write on card charts.

Then you walk down the street to another such facility. As you enter, you are greeted by an elderly woman who looks up from the letter she is writing at the reception desk to smile and ask if she can help. Yes, she assures you, she both lives and works here. You pass a bright gift shop and a coffee shop that is crowded with both white-haired ladies and younger people who push wheelchairs and help the older ones along. These must be the nurses, but their bright clothing and lively manner makes it seem that they are happy granddaughters. Farther on you pass activity rooms and a cafeteria, all clean and well-used. You realize that there must be others here who need a great deal of care, but if all the staff are like those you have seen, you know that residents are living their lives to the fullest extent possible.

Which of these places is where you would like your mother to spend the twilight years of her life? Which would be your choice for yourself? Whenever many of us hear the words "nursing home," we imagine scenes like the first one. But this is unfair, because there are many long-term care facilities that are like the second one. In fact, they vary so much that any attempt to make generalizations is dangerous.

In reality, there are several choices to consider when the health of a spouse or parent begins to fail. These include living with family, living at home with either a family or a professional caregiver, and moving to a long-term care facility. This chapter focuses on making a decision about whether such a facility is appropriate and how to select one. Considering institutional care hardly makes you a maverick. At the present time in North America, between 5 and 9 percent of people over sixty-five live in nursing homes, and the percentage increases with age.

## DEVELOPMENT OF LONG-TERM CARE

The thought of entering a nursing home even as a visitor, let alone as a resident, conjures up sights, sounds and smells that many of us would rather forget. A nursing home can, however, be a godsend for a family or indeed for the individual who could benefit from long-term institutional care.

Many of the negative images and attitudes surrounding modern nursing homes derive from their less-than-pleasant history. The almshouses of the nineteenth century provided not much more than shelter for destitute elderly people. The notion of receiving "care" from such places had not really begun to develop; they were simply asylums where impoverished old people could await their deaths. Until early in this century, there was a very unpleasant social stigma attached to almshouses; they were seen as punishment for having to rely on strangers for shelter, probably the result of an ill-spent life.

According to researchers at the Hastings Center for bioethics, 33 percent of those living in poorhouses in 1880 were elderly. The percentage rose to 66 percent by 1920. There was an accelerating trend for these facilities to be repositories for the old and infirm, places for the burdens of society to go to die.

Between 1920 and the Depression years, mental hospitals seemed to provide a better place for old people suffering from dementia. During the Depression, increasing numbers of elderly people lost their financial self-sufficiency, and the establishment of a social security network finally paved the way for the evolution of the modern nursing home.

Since 1960, nursing homes have been quietly providing excellent care for our aging parents, for the most part; but whenever we hear of them in the media it's because of scandals. These have included charges of negligent care, embezzlement of residents' assets and other unpleasant problems. These unpleasant reports only add to our difficulties in making informed decisions. Clearly, nursing homes suffer from a major image problem.

At the present time, there are over 19,000 nursing homes in the U.S. and over 1,000 in Canada. They have very distinct objectives and provide levels of care that may not be available anywhere else. One objective is to provide care for people who need time to convalesce from illnesses. Acute care facilities — hospitals and clinics — have neither the time, the resources nor the inclination today to care for people beyond the acute phase of their illness. Their concern is to keep patients for as short a time as possible. Long-term care fills in the gap between the acute care hospital and home.

Another role of nursing homes is to provide graduated nursing care for people who suffer from chronic illnesses and whose conditions have deteriorated to the point where they can no longer be independent. In the beginning stages of many chronic conditions such as Parkinson's disease, Alzheimer's disease, advanced arthritis and severe osteoporosis, people are able to continue functioning quite independently and might choose to live at home or in facilities that provide minimal supervision while encouraging continued independence. As the diseases progress, however, they will require care that will have to be increased with the advancement of the disease. Becoming acclimatized to a new facility in the early stages of the disease often makes it easier to cope with the need for increased care later on. For some residents, this need for care progresses to the point where the purpose is to provide terminal, hospice care in contrast to actual treatment for the disease.

Nursing homes can also provide shelter to those aging people who choose not to remain independent and who require a degree of nursing care.

Whatever checkered past nursing homes may have, they have become a necessity as life expectancy increases. As you consider them as an option for aging relatives, remember that there is an important fundamental difference in approach between hospitals and nursing homes. Hospitals exist to provide *treatment*, while nursing homes exist to provide *care*. These two purposes should not be confused as you look for facilities to meet your expectations.

## DEALING WITH YOUR DECISION

No matter how carefully you arrive at the decision in principle for long-term care in a nursing home, you may still find yourself uneasy with it. This is probably a result not of mistrust of yourself, but of the deep-seated societal mistrust of nursing homes, which persists today even though millions of families in North America have experience with good care in these facilities. If you have gathered appropriate information and made a careful decision, you can be assured that you have done the best that you can. If circumstances change, your decision can always be re-evaluated.

One factor that may sway you from your decision in principle is cost. Nursing homes are not cheap, and many people must sign over all their worldly goods to be cared for in these facilities. The annual price tag for nursing home care in the U.S. ranges from U.S. $20,000 to $28,000 per resident, with residents and their families paying 51 percent of the overall costs. In Canada the average is C$32,000 a year. The percentage of the costs that a Canadian resident will have to pay varies depending upon the type of facility, the amount of care that is required and the individual's financial status. How much an individual facility charges and your personal responsibility for the costs are issues that you need to explore while you are making the decision about nursing home care. There is no doubt that cost will be a determining factor in placement, but it should never be the only one.

Before you get to the point of needing such care for yourself, you might investigate long-term care insurance. Many companies in the health insurance business have responded to the upcoming boom in elderly population by offering such insurance, generally for minimum periods of one year of care.

Start by making a broad survey of available facilities in your area and canvassing your friends and relatives for their experiences. Here are some tips for your general investigation:

- Ask lots of questions and prepare as many of them in advance as possible.

- Visit unannounced more than once and observe as much as possible.

- Don't jump at a home just because there is space available.

- Ask your family doctor for his or her opinion.

124

■ Ask the opinions of your friends who have experiences with nursing homes, but remember that they will not be objective assessments.

■ Talk to current residents and their families.

■ Finally, trust your instincts and yourself.

## EVALUATING A NURSING HOME

When you have narrowed the field to just a few candidates, there are many questions that you will be asking yourself and anyone else who might be able to provide you with some insight about the patient's needs and the offerings of each specific facility.

■ How do I know if the care is what the patient wants?

■ How do I know that the care is competent or even better than merely competent?

■ Will the patient be able to see his or her own doctor?

■ Can the facility provide treatment for sudden or serious illness?

■ Will the patient like the people who live there and who work there?

■ Will the patient be able to go out as much as he or she likes?

The list of questions seems endless, and some are of a very personal nature. No one can predict with any degree of accuracy for instance, whether another person will like the people who will become constant companions. But your initial attitudes — yours as a family member, and the attitude of the prospective resident — will have an enormously powerful effect on your reactions to these other questions. If you have made a careful decision about nursing home care and are happy with it in principle, then you can evaluate other factors that are more easily measured, so that you can find a facility that has the best fit for your particular needs.

Here are some areas to explore that will help you to evaluate which facility is best for your needs.

## LEVELS OF CARE PROVIDED

One of the first considerations you will make in selecting a nursing home is what level of care the resident needs now and what the home provides. In addition to present needs, it is wise to consider future needs in light of the resident's general health and any medical conditions that are likely to progress.

At the first, least-intense level of care is a type of facility that is not usually called a nursing home. Rather, it is a facility that provides independent living quarters for seniors who have chosen to leave their homes, often because they are no longer able to maintain the home or would rather not. As the baby boom generation ages, these facilities are likely to increase in number and are likely to provide every level of poshness in their design and facilities. Most urban areas already have many such residences, providing services that are not available to seniors who live in regular apartments or condos. These services include social activities geared to senior groups, educational opportunities, exercise classes, excursions and other innovative ways of providing a full life for older adults. A facility of this nature is for an independent senior who would like to have neighbors of the same generation.

One step above independent living arrangements is care that is designed for those who need only minimal supervision. Facilities at this level often provide apartment-style living with a nurse available to residents twenty-four hours a day. The nurse is responsible for ensuring that residents who are having difficulty, particularly with their medications, have assistance whenever necessary. In addition, these facilities often provide meal service in a central dining room, freeing residents from the extra burden of cooking and then often eating alone. People who are best suited to this level of care are those who can function independently but who feel more comfortable knowing that medical attention is on the premises. People who are in the earliest stages of some chronic conditions, such as Parkinson's disease or difficult-to-control diabetes, will often benefit from the peace of mind this situation can offer.

At a third level is the facility that provides nursing care for people who require assistance for what nurses and doctors call "activities of daily living." These include bathing, dressing, eating, getting exercise and anything else that we usually take for granted in our day-to-day life. In addition to on-the-spot nursing assistance with these activities, these facilities also provide help with medications and supply meals.

Finally, the highest level of care is designed for those individuals who require complete nursing care.

They need someone to do most activities of daily living for them, and they are unable even to get out of bed on their own. Some are more or less confined to bed. People who require this degree of nursing care are often in the final stages of cancer, heart disease, Alzheimer's disease or Parkinson's disease.

This final level of care is the one we most often associate with nursing homes, but each of the other levels of care should also be considered as you choose among options in health care. Some facilities house some or all of these levels under one roof. These would be particularly good choices for patients suffering from a disease that will require increasing levels of nursing care. The multi-level facility would also be ideal for couples who may require different levels of care but who choose to enter a nursing home together. They can live under the same roof and see one another easily every day.

## RATIO OF CAREGIVERS TO RESIDENTS

Are there enough staff members to give the care needed by the residents? We have heard it said that you can judge a hospital or nursing home by how long you have to wait for a bedpan. This may be an oversimplification, but the test may finally come down to something this fundamental.

It is very difficult to make this assessment directly unless you have lived in the facility yourself, but some indirect measures are possible. Ask whether the facility has received endorsement or accreditation from an outside body. This means that the home has been assessed by an impartial third party against objective standards. You might also ask how many residents are under the care of one worker; the appropriateness of this ratio depends wholly on the level of care that is supposed to be provided. It would be helpful to take a friend who is a nurse (not a doctor) along with you when you visit to ask these questions. A nursing background allows a much more useful evaluation.

In addition, since you are likely to visit during the day, ask about the number of staff on at night. Needing help to go to the bathroom doesn't stop at 7:00 p.m.

## RATIO OF REGISTERED NURSES TO NON-PROFESSIONAL STAFF

In addition to asking about the absolute number of staff available at any one time, you should ask how many of these are registered nurses, licensed practical nurses, registered (or certified) nursing assistants, personal care workers or untrained aides. The duties of the registered nurses — the professional staff members — are mandated by law. The licensed practical nurses (LPNs) and registered nursing assistants (RNAs) are also licensed, but their responsibilities often differ by institution. In hospitals LPNs and RNAs are often not permitted to perform certain duties, such as administering medications, but this is often a requirement in nursing homes. Ask whether the staff members giving out medications have received enough extra training for the job.

Personal care workers are generally trained by

short courses to provide very basic care such as bathing, dressing, toileting and feeding. Nurses' aides are often untrained. In some facilities they seem to provide some actual nursing care; in other situations they can only deliver water, help the other staff to make beds and lift patients and provide general clean-up.

An acute care hospital will have much more professional staff than non-professional staff; it is usually the opposite in a nursing home. Don't expect the level of education and training of the staff here to be the same as in a hospital. This would be neither cost-effective nor necessary for the levels of care required.

## NUTRITION AND ACTIVITY PROGRAMS

Although you shouldn't expect that the food in a nursing home will rival that of the finest restaurants in town, it should be presented properly (it should be appropriately hot or cold) and it should be nutritious. Inquire about the credentials of the person supervising the selection of the menu and the food service; it should be a nutritionist, although this person may not be a full-time staff member. Good-quality supervision will ensure that health and safety precautions are observed. Your best approach to evaluating this aspect of a nursing home is to eat there.

The home should also have a planned activity program for residents. If the residents simply sit and watch television all day every day, they have certainly lost something of their human dignity. Ask about daily and weekly activity programs and who runs them. Many facilities have recreation professionals in charge of the programs, while others use the services of volunteers. Volunteers might not provide the ideal situation, but they can operate programs that are stimulating and interesting for the participants.

## ACCESS TO PERSONAL PHYSICIANS

The number of specialists in the care of the elderly is growing, but family physicians still provide the primary care for people in nursing homes. Although you might wish to have the resident's own family doctor continue as his or her personal physician, this may not be possible. Usually the difficulty is simply that the nursing home is too far from the physician's usual territory. Clearly it is too much to ask of a doctor to visit regularly in a remote location where he or she probably has only one patient.

So you may need to check out the facility's own physician. This person will usually be the facility's medical director; in addition to providing care to residents, he or she is responsible for the administrative aspects of the medical care in the home. The responsibilities of the physician attending to patients in a long-term care facility are generally agreed to be:

- deciding about any appropriate medical care that the resident may require, including the ordering and monitoring of medications;

- monitoring the resident at regular intervals;

- discussing the resident's condition with the nursing staff and family whenever necessary;

- maintaining the resident's medical records;

131

- consulting with specialist physicians as necessary;
- respecting the policies of the facility.

If the patient's own doctor is prepared to continue care, determine the facility's policies regarding the attendance of outside physicians.

## FOLLOWING UP

Don't make the mistake of assuming that your role in a family member's health care decisions is over once he or she has entered the nursing home. The process and context in a nursing home are quite different than at home or even in a hospital, but there are still decisions to be made.

Your family member may be competent upon entering the home, but the simple fact of aging suggests his or her competence will decline. Three-quarters of people in nursing homes are over seventy-five, and with the inevitable chronic conditions of aging, nursing home residents are likely to have more difficulty with independent decision-making. The sooner you can help the resident to determine his or her overall attitude toward health care, and to communicate it to you and the health care staff, the better. Just like other older adults, nursing home residents should be encouraged to do some advance planning for specific health care decisions as well.

In the nursing home, the professional nursing staff have more responsibility and accountability than they would in a hospital. The nurses play a much larger role in decisions here than in hospitals, largely because physicians do not see their patients on a daily basis, often not even on a weekly basis. Doctors rely on the nurses' observations and recommendations here even more than they would in an acute care facility.

What this means for residents and family members is that you need to get to know the nursing staff. They need to know how you feel about difficult care decisions so that they can convey this perspective to the physician if the resident is unable to do so and the family can't be reached. From your first evaluative visit to such a facility, start to familiarize yourself with these valuable allies in the resident's care.

One final note is worth considering here. The people who choose to work in long-term care tend to have a different perspective on health and illness than do those who choose the more acute, often apparently high-powered settings. These differences are reflected, at least to a degree, in the way the nursing homes react to crises that often develop in the conditions of the residents. Crises tend not to be the all-out dramas that we see depicted in hospital shows on television. Generally, nursing homes are not equipped with either the machinery or the personnel necessary to give the kind of care that would be available in the emergency room of a hospital, so treatment of these crises is often dictated by the resources.

With current concerns about cost containment in hospitals, however, sicker patients are being discharged from acute care settings to long-term care facilities. This trend has resulted in many long-term care facilities becoming better equipped than they used to be. Find out what facilities are available, how they will be used, who will use them and what are the procedures for dealing with emergencies and transfer to acute care settings.

Seeing a family member through the process of moving into a nursing home may lead you to think more about your own future. It may be your hope that you not become a personal burden to your own children. As one patient put it, "I don't want to ruin their lives. They shouldn't put up with me. Put me in a home." If this reflects your own perspective, tell your family now. If you become incapacitated and are unable to make decisions for yourself, they can do as you wished. Relieving them of unnecessary guilt may be the best legacy you can leave behind.

# 9 Home Care

SHARON J., FORTY-SIX, is a high school teacher and the mother of an active preschooler. She has her hands full. Old enough to think of themselves as "older adults," she and her husband delayed parenthood until their careers were well established and they no longer had to worry about financial concerns. But now they have joined the "sandwich generation," caring both for a young child and for Sharon's aging mother, a seventy-year-old widow with advancing Alzheimer's disease. Sharon herself coordinates her mother's care, but she has hired a nursing assistant from an agency to provide for the actual requirements, which involve helping her mother each day with bathing, dressing, going to the bathroom and eating, as well as providing companionship. Theirs is a busy household, with a nanny also coming daily to care for Sharon's preschooler. At the end of the day, Sharon is often too exhausted to sleep. She is not alone.

This morning she is having coffee with two friends who are also caring for aging parents. Their situations are, however, all different. Sonja V. is forty-two years old and is the primary caregiver for her elderly father. He is almost eighty and has terminal cancer. He is completely bedridden. Twice a week a volunteer with the respite program of the local cancer society comes to her home for two hours. This is Sonja's cue to race out of the house to do grocery shopping and banking and, on a rare occasion, to get her hair cut or have coffee with friends. Hers is also a twenty-four-hour-a-day job. She never complains. Sonja knows, however, that her father does not have much longer to live, and she has every intention of making him as comfortable as possible, "as he has always done for me," she says.

Ann H.'s mother has recently moved in with Ann and her family. Unable to take care of her own home any longer, Ann's mother had spent some time deciding against nursing home care. Over the protestations of her husband and her three teen-aged children, Ann had offered to have her mother move in with them. Her mother does not need nursing care and is quite safe to be left alone for periods of time, but she is very demanding, and Ann often feels as though she is a child again, always having to do as Mother wishes.

Some of these are happy stories, and some are not. But they do reflect a certain reality of today's North America. It has been estimated that there may be up to three older people cared for in family homes for every one in an institutional setting. These statistics are difficult to verify, as home care is not necessarily known outside the home. For a variety of reasons, home care (not only of the elderly) is the fastest-growing area of the health care delivery systems in both Canada and the U.S.

Economics are frequently at the root of this growth. As acute care has become increasingly complex, technologically oriented and expensive, there has been a movement across the continent to discharge patients from hospitals as early as possible. These people are not always able to cope on their own, but the home makes a more cost-effective setting in which to provide whatever care they need.

Home care is not a modern phenomenon. In fact, medicine has been practiced in the home for centuries. Doctors were making house calls and delivering their care in homes when hospitals were still looked upon as places to go to die. So the modern trend is actually a return to where health care began.

## EXAMINING YOUR DECISION

If you have concluded that home care is the best solution to the health care needs of your parent or spouse, you need to examine why you have opted for this choice. Caring for an aging person in the home can be very stressful for the modern North American family. Many of us are not ready for it, but that does not mean that it is not a reasonable choice. It can actually be a very rewarding experience, as many family caregivers will attest. You just have to be as sure as you can be.

If, for example, you have decided that you will care for your aging mother in your home as opposed to placing her in a nursing home, you need to ask yourself a few important questions. Here are some suggestions to begin your re-examination of your decision:

- Are you aware that taking care of someone at home can produce three major sources of stress: physical, emotional and lifestyle?

- Have you realistically examined your own capabilities, both physically and emotionally?

- Are you prepared to change your lifestyle?

- Whose needs are you putting first: your own needs or your parent's needs?

First, as you examine whether you are being realistic about the level of stress that you can cope with, you need to determine if you have the physical stamina. How much stamina you will need to cope successfully depends upon how much care the person needs now and in future and how much outside help you will have. Even if you are not going to give the actual care yourself, outside caregivers are often not available around the clock. You will certainly have some degree of physical involvement. If you are the one who will be giving the actual physical care to a loved one, the physical commitment can be overwhelming. Only recently have researchers begun to look at the long-term effects of physical stress on wives and daughters who give this kind of care (it is well known that most family caregivers are women).

Your emotional stress level depends largely upon the pre-existing relationships that you have developed: your relationships with the family member who requires care, with other people who will be living in the household and with outside support networks. If these relationships are already sources of emotional stress, home care may make matters worse.

You may not have considered what we are calling lifestyle stress. If you are not used to having an older member of your family around, this can have an effect on the lifestyle that you have come to cherish. You may have to reconsider how you spend your vacations, what entertaining you do, whether your children can have noisy friends over, how many business trips you can take and so on. Take a close look at the elements of your lifestyle that you are not willing to change; if these are likely to be affected by your decision to be a home caregiver, your lifestyle stress is likely to escalate considerably.

After you have looked at some of the realities of your decision, go back to see if you can honestly determine whose needs you are putting first. It may seem to you that you are placing the needs of the person who requires care before your own. While this would be noble, it may not be true. People choose to care for loved ones for a variety of reasons. You may have a real need to give something back to a parent: that is your own need, not your parent's. You may feel guilty about the lifestyle you have chosen (or any one of a dozen other things grown children feel guilty about) and wish to make it up to a parent: that is also your own need. None of these reasons is either bad or good, they just need to be recognized for what they are and faced. Once you face the truth of your motives, then you can decide if you are willing to live with them.

The decision to give care in the family home means different things to different people. The range of care that may be required and given is vast. The care might include any of the following:

- provision of companionship

- shopping assistance

- transportation

- homemaking

- assistance with personal care (bathing, grooming, dressing)

- administration of medications

- administration of medical treatments (oxygen, dressing changes)

- physiotherapy or occupational therapy

- complete nursing care for a bedridden patient

Make a simple list of the care required now and the care that is likely to be needed at various intervals in the future, so you can begin to develop a realistic picture of what you will need to provide that care in your household. Then list everything you will need, from furniture to the kind and amount of outside help. Be as specific as possible. Your family may be able to help with many of the items on your needs list, but some require professional help. In addition, even if a family caregiver can handle each of the tasks individually, the sheer number of responsibilities may be more than you can be expected to cope with on your own.

## ASSESSING YOUR PHYSICAL SURROUNDINGS

Family homes are not the same as institutions designed and built with older people in mind. They are designed for able-bodied, independent people. Consider the modifications that you have to make when you bring a new baby into the home. While the child is young, you find yourself living with electrical outlet covers that you invariably forget about until you have tried unsuccessfully to ram a plug into one; you add unsightly but useful gates at the tops and bottoms of all staircases, childproof (and often adult-proof) catches on cupboards and other safety precautions. Clearly, our homes were not made for toddlers. In the same way, our homes are usually not completely ready for aging people, who may have difficulty with mobility and judgement. You may need to make some modifications in your physical surroundings.

Is your home owned or rented? This is vitally important if you will be faced with the possibility of making any physical adjustments. Some landlords may not object to adding a wheelchair ramp to an outside entrance or knocking down walls to enlarge doorways, but others will balk at the suggestion of something as simple as attaching a handrail on the wall next to the toilet.

Once you have explored the extent to which you have permission to alter the physical surroundings, assess whether alterations are feasible. If stairs are likely to be a problem, look at the location of some primary rooms in the home, namely the bedroom, the bathroom and the kitchen. Will you be able to minimize the need for using the stairs? Can a room on the main floor be used as a bedroom? If stairs are going to be a fact of life, will you be able to add a device for assisting with their use, such as a lift?

Much of your assessment of the physical surroundings will be based on the current and future physical condition of your family member and the level of care that the condition demands. One other important consideration is the degree of independence that the aging person wants. If the aging person living alone will be preparing meals, for example, you need to ensure that conditions like arthritis of the fingers do not deprive him or her of the ability to do simple things like open cans. An occupational therapist can help to develop devices so that your relative can maintain some independence.

## WHO WILL GIVE THE CARE?

One of the most difficult decisions that you will have to make is who will actually be giving the care. Because of the age segregation of our society, the decision to care for an aging person in the family home is not a simple continuation of a well-established lifestyle. It is often a major change for all parties involved. Although most family caregivers today are women, this is not a role that all women fall into naturally, particularly given the number of responsibilities that most women today have outside the home.

So you have two real options in caregiving right from the start: the care can be provided by a family member or by someone hired for that purpose. In some cases a blend of the two can provide a third option.

## FAMILY CAREGIVERS

People choose family caregivers for a variety of reasons, one of the most obvious being economic. It can be very costly to hire someone for this purpose. Even if finances push you into this decision, consider these important questions.

- Do you have the physical capability to give the needed care?

- Will you be able to give knowledgeable, safe care?

- Do you have the commitment to alter your lifestyle as necessary?

- Will you be willing to reassess this decision at some point in the future when circumstances (family life, career demands, level of care required) change?

- If you do not do this, will you have lost an opportunity?

Not everyone is ready, willing or able to give this much of themselves, and you should not feel guilty about saying no. Furthermore, not every parent or spouse *wants* home care, even if you offer it. Make sure you discuss this openly before you make a well-meaning mistake.

Many people see caregiving as an opportunity for personal growth. As nurse Sharon Fish says in her book about caring for a loved one with Alzheimer's disease, "It can make us more courageous, more compassionate and more patient people."

If this is your choice, remember that you are not alone. North American statistics indicate that 80 percent of all days of home care are provided by family members. There are some support groups that might make dealing with the stress a little easier.

## HIRING OUTSIDE HELP

If your personal preference, the level of care required and your finances lead you to choose outside help, keep an important fact in mind. Even if you hire someone to give the care, the coordination of the care falls to a member of the family. In addition, unless you have twenty-four-hour-a-day assistance, there will be times when the actual care will also fall to a family caregiver.

Your first step in finding suitable help is to define exactly what you want this person to do. Sit down and put your requirements in writing. List all the care that is required; then consider the extent to which this person will be involved. If, for example, you indicate that you will need help with meals, what does this entail? Does it mean setting up a tray and feeding, or does it also include meal preparation or grocery shopping? Does helping with personal grooming also mean doing the laundry? Take every activity and extend it to all its related activities to determine your expectations.

Next consider how often you need to have the person in the home. Is this a daily requirement, or twice weekly? Will it be for two hours at a time or twelve? Will it be feasible or even desirable for the caregiver to live in the home?

Then start thinking about the kind of person that would fit well into your family situation. Would you prefer someone older and more experienced, or younger and perhaps more energetic? Apart from technical requirements related to the level of care, consider the qualifications that you believe would be most appropriate. Do you believe that you need a registered nurse, or would a nursing assistant, personal care worker or homemaker be just as valuable to you? How much do you plan to pay for this care?

The answers to these questions will give you the basis for developing a job description. Just as large organizations have written job descriptions for their employees, you too will be an employer and will need one as well. It will clearly point out to the employee the duties for which he or she has been contracted to perform and that you have contracted to pay for. This will help both in the hiring process and in later disputes that may arise about obligations. A sample job description is on page 151.

Now, what method will you use to find this person or persons? You might ask people you know to recommend workers, but this is probably not a broad enough search. The two basic choices you have to begin your search are to go to an employment agency, pay their fee and have them find you an appropriate person; or to put an advertisement in the paper. Both options have their attractions and their drawbacks.

One of your first thoughts might be to place an advertisement in the local paper. This is certainly cheap and can be effective. The main drawback is the long, circuitous route that you will probably have to follow to get from that cheap ad to your final decision about who you will hire. Depending upon what qualifications you are seeking, you may be inundated with applications. Many of these will be totally inappropriate for your family situation, but you may not be able to discern that without dozens of interviews. Even then, you may be left wondering about the qualifications and references of some of the applicants. If you have both the time and the inclination to meet these candidates and follow up, you may find, as many others have, that you like the results.

The other approach is to hire through an employment agency. Try to select an agency based on personal recommendation by someone that you trust. This may be a friend, a neighbor, a co-worker or your doctor. To use an agency you must pay a finder's fee, which can sometimes be quite expensive; but if you are a busy person and can swing it, will probably be well worth the investment. Look for an agency that will not charge you a second fee if the first worker you hire does not work out within the first three months.

The agency will want to see, probably in writing, your job description. They will need some sense of your time requirements and how much you are willing to pay. A placement counsellor will interview you to try to determine both your requirements and your wishes. The agency will then try to match your needs with an appropriate person who is looking for a job. They will have already checked the references, but it is still your responsibility to do so for yourself and we recommend that you do not overlook this. Using an agency will reduce the number of actual interviews that you will have to conduct.

Both of these options will result in your being the

actual employer. In these situations, you will be required to conduct all business transactions, including payment of salary, negotiation of vacation time and sick leave, directly with your employee. If this person is late for work, you will have to deal with it directly. You may be quite happy to do this, or you may prefer to have someone else responsible for such things. In the latter case, you will be more comfortable not hiring an individual but contracting with a home care agency to provide you with help.

## HOME CARE AGENCIES

Home care agencies are springing up all over North America. They provide a wide variety of levels of service, from homemaking to sophisticated nursing care. When you engage the services of an agency, they send the workers to you but maintain complete employer-employee relations with them. You pay your fees to the agency, which, in turn, pays the employee. If there is a disciplinary problem, the agency will deal with it. If you have complaints about the individual, you can tell the individual's supervisor and that person will deal with it.

There is, of course, a price to be paid for this service. You do relinquish some control, and it costs more. Obviously, the agency has to get its cut for doing all the regular paperwork as well as clinical supervision. Reputable agencies do, however, also provide ongoing education for their employees, and some offer stepped care, if you require such an approach. With stepped care, if your care requirements increase and the worker you have can no longer provide the new level of care, the agency will simply send someone with more appropriate qualifications.

There is no question that having a total stranger come into your home to provide care for a loved one can be stressful. Any mother who has hired a new nanny to care for a child can attest to that. But when you are able to find someone who is a good "fit," the benefits to you, your family and the person receiving care can be incredible.

## RESPITE CARE

Whether the caregiver is a family member or an employee, you will probably need respite care at one time or another. The term "respite" means "a temporary intermission of labor" or "an interval of rest." In law, the term means a reprieve. In home care, all of these apply. Respite care gives you the opportunity to be temporarily relieved of some of the constant stress of having a loved one in your home who requires care.

If you have chosen to provide family caregiving, consider what will happen over a period of time if you are unable to get out of the house even for a few hours of personal errands. Perhaps all you need is two hours to read a book and relax. Being a family caregiver means being on duty twenty-four hours a day, except when someone else takes over the duties. Your responsibility to yourself dictates that you make arrangements for respite — even though it may take some effort and creativity.

What will happen to that trip to Disney World that you have been promising your young children for some time? When will you ever get the opportunity to go if your family member needs your care? Even if you have someone coming into your home to give the care, it is unlikely that this person's own family obligations will allow him or her to simply move in for the two weeks of your vacation. Perhaps the time you need isn't even for a vacation but to attend a work-related conference or a family wedding or funeral out of town. You will need to investigate your options well in advance.

Most cities today have some kind of respite care services available for these situations. The simplest services consist of a force of volunteers who will come to your home for a few hours once or twice a week to provide companionship and ensure safety. They do not give care of any sort, but they allow the primary caregiver to do other things.

The next level of care is often provided by agencies who will send experienced individuals to your home for longer periods of time, from a weekend to a couple of weeks. These people will carry out all the required activities, providing the family with much-needed respite.

Another form of respite care that might be more attractive to you does not require you to have a stranger come into your home. This service is provided by some long-term care facilities that have units devoted to short-term residents. The person requiring care will go the facility for that short period of time and then return home. If everyone is to be comfortable with this alternative, it must be well understood. The person who is going to the facility needs to understand as far as possible that this is only a temporary arrangement. If you intend this short-term care to be a prelude to a longer-term arrangement, be straightforward about it.

As you look at the alternatives in respite care, examine your own family situation and your physical facilities to determine the option that is most appropriate for you and most affordable. Information about local respite facilities can be obtained from your local offices of voluntary organizations that provide services to older adults. Organizations that support patients with particular diseases — such as Alzheimer's societies and cancer associations — may also be helpful.

Would you want home care for yourself, if your future needs call for it? Considering it today and discussing it with your family could ease their minds at a later date. Your thinking on this topic should also be brought into your financial planning for your retirement years.

Even with the best-laid plans, you may not have the luxury of this option for care in your later years, but if you begin to think about it before it becomes a reality, you may open more doors. If you do make a decision that you would prefer to be cared for in your own home as you age, you are certainly going to find that you are in good company. Baby boomers have always relished control over their own lives, and this is likely to continue in the next century with more and more of them opting to stay in their homes and have the caregivers come to them.

# SAMPLE JOB DESCRIPTION FOR AN IN-HOME CAREGIVER

## The Position

This position for a personal care worker for Mrs. H. is designed to provide a high level of comfort and safety in everyday activities, thus contributing to Mrs. H.'s quality of life.

## The Duties

1. Assistance with all personal hygiene activities including bathing, dressing, grooming and toileting.

2. Meal preparation following a nutrition guide provided by the family.

3. Meal serving and assistance with eating.

4. Daily companionship including activities such as reading, listening to music, puzzles and other activities that might be suggested by Mrs. H. or her daughter from time to time.

5. Assistance with exercise, outside when weather permits.

6. Assuring safety at all times.

7. Administration of medications that have been poured by Mrs. H.'s daughter.

8. General tidying of Mrs. H.'s rooms and ensuring that materials are cleaned up after use.

## Accountability

This position is accountable to Mrs. H.'s daughter, who will be the employer. At no time is Mrs. H. to be left alone.

# PART FOUR

# Making
# Final
# Decisions

# 10 Death and Dying

A WISE MAN once said: "There is one path for all, but each must walk it in his own way." We come now to that path which includes the one experience that all human beings have in common: we will all die some day. The older we get, the closer that day comes. But none of us is likely to see or feel the experience in quite the same way. Modern health care is far and away the most important contributor to the fact that there are so many different ways to have this experience today.

Human beings have always been concerned about living a long life. As we approach the end of the twentieth century and the bulging population wave heads toward older adulthood, concern about aging has never had a higher profile. Just walk into any store that sells magazines and take a few moments to browse among the multitude of publications that provide their readers with information designed to make them healthy and live longer. And people buy them by the hundreds of thousands.

In North America today, we have developed a bone-chilling fear of death. The reality is, however, that immortality is a myth and death is a fact of everyone's life. Once you have accepted that, you can move on to the realization that part of the fear lies with a feeling of powerlessness that we don't cherish. It is clear that we want control over the way we live, so it hardly seems odd that we also want control over issues that relate to our deaths. Knowledge and forethought are empowering in general and no less so when we use them to exercise control over the end of our lives.

Even though medical science has already extended North American life expectancy by 30 or more years since the beginning of this century, we remain obsessed with stretching it still further. Researchers have attempted to estimate how much longer we could realistically hope to extend human lives by eliminating some chronic diseases. Some suggest that elimination of all types of cancers would increase life expectancy for men by three years; and if ischemic heart disease (the kind that narrows arteries and causes heart attacks) were no longer a problem, men could add on about another three and a half years. If we could get rid of heart disease, cancer and diabetes, men could expect to live just over fifteen years longer.

But elimination of these acute illnesses that cause our so-called premature deaths would not give us immortality. What it would give us is, to a large extent, a miserable existence. Those extra years would most likely be marked by crippling diseases that would be the focus of our existence. Alzheimer's disease, osteoporosis, arthritis and a host of other diseases that are more frequent in old people would reduce the quality of those years. It seems, then, that quantity of life is often at the expense of its quality.

Perhaps the first step toward gaining control over our dying is to stop thinking about it in such negative terms and recognize that there can be something comforting about the thought of a good death at the end of a good life. Start exploring your feelings, accept them — and get ready to make some important decisions.

## WHAT IS "DEATH" IN MODERN MEDICINE?

This may seem like a very odd question to you, but modern medical technology has made it necessary for us to examine its answer before we can make any decisions about what we want and what we do not want. Death has not really changed; only the way that we define its arrival in medical terms has.

In days gone by, people died at home, not in a hospital. They were surrounded by loved ones and familiar spaces rather than an array of white-coated strangers and pulsating, bleeping and dripping equipment. The notion of a dignified death is a modern creation, as a response to all the technological advances that have decreased the dignity of this very human event.

When all the doctor could do was hold the patient's hand and hope that his or her presence might calm the family, people slipped quietly into death. Although that can still happen today if a person dies at home, a large proportion of North

Americans die in hospitals. In fact, between 75 and 80 percent of all deaths on this continent occur in hospitals. That makes it a high probability that you too will die in a hospital, unless you have made other special arrangements.

Walter H. was an eighty-year-old man who had been diagnosed some time earlier with terminal cancer. He had been admitted to the intensive care unit of his community hospital because he now needed constant, sophisticated nursing care. It is likely that he would not have been admitted to the ICU in a larger, busier, urban hospital, but his admission was not so unusual in a smaller facility.

Several days after his admission to the unit, Walter suffered a cardiac arrest in the middle of the day. When his heart monitor stopped bleeping, the nurses sprang into action and he was resuscitated. Before the day shift of nurses left for home, the scene repeated itself. When the night nurses arrived, one of the interns doing a community hospital rotation poked his head around the corner and said, "We're stealing them from the Lord. If Mr. H. arrests tonight, try to resuscitate him, but don't try too hard."

At 6:30 the next morning, Walter died. He had never regained consciousness since the first arrest.

Does this really happen in hospitals? It certainly does. It happens every day of every week in most hospitals across the continent. The problem here is the one we posed earlier. When did Walter really die? Before you can really make a decision about how you want to be treated yourself, you need to understand how health professionals view this issue.

There was a time when death was defined as cardiac arrest: the individual stops breathing and his or her heart stops beating. But modern methods of cardiopulmonary resuscitation (CPR) have changed all that. A physician used to place his or her ear on the chest of the patient and, hearing no heartbeat and feeling no breath upon his or her cheek, declare the patient dead. Today, when a cardiac arrest happens in a location where someone, not necessarily a physician, knows how to administer CPR, an attempt will usually be made to "bring the patient back." CPR is the application of external heart massage and ventilation (breathing) so that blood may continue to be pumped through the person's body, carrying oxygen, until the heart and lungs resume operations on their own.

By definition, then, death must be something different than cardiac arrest. Since we now know that people are not necessarily dead just because their hearts have stopped, we recognize that it is the death of the brain that signifies the real end of life. The brain does not die until about ten minutes after cardiac arrest, so medical and nursing personnel in an acute care setting typically feel compelled to take action in that interval to restart hearts and prevent brain death.

With older patients, however, is this automatic response the wisest one? The most important concern must be the degree of success of these procedures. Researchers define a successful resuscitation effort as being one in which the patient lives to be discharged from hospital. Using this definition, studies have shown overall success rates varying from as little as zero to as much as 30 percent. In one study of people over seventy who had suffered cardiac arrest, 22 percent survived initially after CPR but fewer than 4 percent survived to hospital discharge. Of these few survivors, some were seriously injured by the resuscitation itself.

Defining death is not an academic discussion. It has a real impact on how older patients are treated in hospitals today. Clearly there are choices and decisions to be made. If you do not want to leave those decisions to others when your own death is near, give some thought now to the options you may have.

## FOREGOING LIFE-SUSTAINING TREATMENT

As discussed earlier, among the decisions you have the right to make is a decision to refuse treatment. Even at the point where refusal of treatment means death, you retain that right. For health professionals, though, your refusal presents a greater ethical dilemma when your life is at stake, because it may conflict with their sense that they have a duty to treat you and with their belief in the sanctity of life. Nevertheless the notion that vegetative life should be maintained at all costs is losing ground.

Life-sustaining treatments include antibiotic therapy, artificial ventilation, artificial pacing of the heart, dialysis for kidney failure, and some kinds of surgery. Feeding, by natural or artificial means, is also life-sustaining, although some health professionals may not consider it a "treatment." Sometimes, however, people get to a point where they do not want any further treatment for an illness, and nourishment is sustaining a life that they no longer want sustained.

As long as it is not just a comfort measure, we consider feeding a treatment that you have the right to refuse, just as you might refuse to have any more chemotherapy for your cancer. Be warned, however, that hospital administrators do not like the idea of patients "starving" to death while in their care (see pages 95-96). Although this view is technically incorrect — if you are terminally ill, it is your disease to which you succumb — it may be persuasive to your caregivers, and you will need to be firm and clear if this is the option you choose.

## "DO NOT RESUSCITATE" ORDERS

A DNR order is a medical order placed on the patient's chart to indicate that CPR is not to be administered if the patient has a cardiac arrest. In other words, the patient is to be allowed to die peacefully. The order is given for terminally ill patients, following discussion, if at all possible, with the patient and the family.

Today this option seems to make good sense, although health professionals went through years of debates about whether DNR orders are ethical or legal. It was not uncommon in the past for terminally ill patients to be subjected to futile attempts at resuscitation without any consultation with their families. It is still difficult for some health professionals to ignore their elaborate equipment and their arsenal of emergency drugs in favor of letting the patient's disease process take its course. They believe they are not doing their job if they do not do everything medically possible. In fact, many believed and continue to believe they would be leaving themselves open to a lawsuit if they did not attempt resuscitation in all cases.

Most hospitals still have a policy that, unless a DNR order is specifically made, resuscitation will be attempted. If the physician does not raise the subject with the patient or the family, even when the patient is near death, the order will probably not go on the chart. The nurses are the people most likely to discover that a patient has "arrested" and, since they are not in a position to make a medical decision about whether or not to resuscitate, they are obliged by hospital policy to do so.

If you want to give the medical and nursing staff this option, you may have to bring up the subject yourself with your doctor. You will have to ask the question: What will you do if I have a cardiac arrest? If you do want to be resuscitated, make certain the doctors and nurses know this is your wish. If, on the other hand, you do not want this procedure, ensure that such an order is written by your doctor and added to your chart.

When in doubt, medical personnel are more likely to err on the side of resuscitating. Sometimes, on the other hand, doctors and nurses may be inclined to forgo the procedure but find that the family is demanding resuscitation even when the situation is hopeless and the procedure is "medically futile." In other words, there is no medical reason to hope that the effort will be successful.

Why a family may request such a futile procedure is as unique as the family. It may result from a feeling of guilt that they have not done everything possible to prevent the death. It may result from a deep-seated fear of death, or there may be other self-serving reasons, such as an inability to face the loss. Embedded in these inappropriate requests is a lack of understanding about how harmful CPR might actually be to the patient; there is a risk of broken ribs or brain damage, even with the best quality of care. It may, in fact, prolong not the person's life, but his or her dying. When someone suffers from a medical condition for which CPR would offer no medical benefit, it is irresponsible to ask health care workers to carry out a futile procedure.

A DNR order is not supposed to change any other aspect of the patient's care. Even though patients and families have decided that CPR will not be needed, that does not mean that they have given up any other treatment, unless that is specifically decided upon. These orders are reviewed regularly and can be cancelled as conditions change or as the patient requests. You and your family should find out how often these orders are reviewed and who reviews them.

## SUICIDE AND ASSISTED SUICIDE

Lately the media have followed the controversies surrounding suicide machines and the publication of specific instructions about how to take your own life. There is little doubt that, like the abortion debate, the issue of an individual's right to take his or her own life polarizes the population into those who believe that each of us has the right to determine our own fates and those who believe that only God or other deities have that right. Most of us are probably somewhere in the middle, wondering whether suicide might be something to consider in certain circumstances.

As a cause of death, suicide ranks in the top ten. Although adults over sixty-five account for only 11 to 12 percent of the North American population, they account for about one-quarter of all suicides. Suicide is more common in men, those who live alone, those who have recently lost a spouse, and those who have suffered from an illness or a physical change. The question here is: Is suicide a reasonable alternative for some people with terminal illness?

Do you have the right to take your own life if you have decided that death is preferable to living with a specific medical condition? On the whole, society seems to say you do not, although the philosophers continue their debate. Negative messages about suicide are everywhere, and suicide intervention centers are found throughout North America. The consensus seems to be that suicide is something to be prevented, something that only insane or at least severely maladjusted people would do.

There is, however, growing support for the position that paternalism in health care is misguided. As we age, we make serious decisions about our own health; and realistically, one of those decisions is whether to continue living with a medical condition that cannot be changed and is seriously compromising our quality of life. Garnering support for this

164

decision, however, may be easier said than done. Without considerable education, both family doctors and families often have difficulty accepting a suicide decision; the usual reaction is to conclude that the patient is no longer competent.

Taking your own life may be a simple matter of making a plan and following it. If, however, you wish to end your life but are physically unable to do it yourself, that is quite a different matter. Engaging someone to help is called assisted suicide. You may find a sympathetic doctor or nurse, but the issue poses such difficult ethical dilemmas for health professionals that it is more likely to be a family member.

In 1985 journalist Betty Rollin related the story of how she assisted her seventy-six-year-old mother, who suffered from terminal cancer, to end her life. Her book *Last Wish* chronicles both the mechanics of the act and its ethics. At the end, as the medications begin to work, Rollin's mother says, "Remember, I am the most happy woman. And this is my wish." Her loving daughter ends the book with this: "I know that she has found the door she was looking for and that it has closed, gently, behind her." Although it seems difficult to argue with the peace that this act gave both mother and daughter, assisting someone with a suicide remains an illegal act in most jurisdictions.

## EUTHANASIA

It seems ironic that the word "euthanasia," which invites such heated debate among health professionals and others, should have its roots in the Greek for "a good death." In fact, dictionaries define euthanasia as "a painless peaceful death" or "deliberately putting to death painlessly of a person suffering from a terminal disease," a synonym is "mercy-killing." In the medical literature, euthanasia is generally subdivided to differentiate between "active" and "passive euthanasia" and between "voluntary" and "involuntary euthanasia."

Active euthanasia is ending an individual's life by actively administering something that will accomplish this goal. This differs from assisted suicide, as the act is carried out not by the person who wishes to end his or her life, but by someone else. It also differs from "passive euthanasia," which is sometimes equated with respecting the individual's right to refuse therapy. Although no specific act to end the person's life is carried out, by not administering therapy, the medical personnel are, in effect, involved in the ending of a life.

Euthanasia is "voluntary" when the individual whose life is in question makes the voluntary choice to end it. It is "involuntary" when someone else makes that choice. It is this latter issue that is of greatest concern to those who debate ethical issues, because of the problems that could occur if others begin to decide who will live and who will die.

This discussion is confined to situations where you have decisions to make. In other words, we are dealing with the issue of voluntary, active euthanasia. Strictly speaking, it is illegal in North America, and anyone who helps carry out your wishes could face criminal charges. But in fact, active euthanasia occurs throughout North America. The practice of "snowing" terminally ill cancer patients with increasing doses of painkillers, with the full knowledge of their effects on respiration and consciousness, has been going on in hospitals for years. In a recent University of Colorado study of physicians, fully one-third said that they had, in fact, given painkillers that they knew sped up the time of death.

Many professionals and lay people now support the notion that competent adults who are terminally ill ought to have the right to engage the services of a health professional to end their lives if they so choose. In 1991, however, when voters in the state of Washington were given the opportunity to indicate if they wanted to have the right to ask their physicians to help them die, 54 percent said no. On the other hand, 46 percent voted for it, and this is considerable support. One of the groups that opposed the law was the state medical society. Its position, like that of other physicians' groups, is that the law would place doctors in an unwelcome position, in conflict with their primary goal of preserving life.

Even if you believe you have the right to active euthanasia so that you may exercise control over where and when you will die, and even if you believe it is the moral thing to do under specific circumstances, be warned: euthanasia is currently illegal in every jurisdiction in both the United States and Canada. From a legal point of view, this is not a decision you have the right to make.

## A DIGNIFIED DEATH?

Is it at all possible for a death to be dignified? Some people think not. We believe, however, that death is as much a part of being human as birth is. It is the final chapter in the story of each of our lives. If ours has been a good biography, then death should be a fitting conclusion. One cannot, however, make a poor book into a good one simply by making the last chapter longer. There is such a thing as knowing when to quit.

The term "dignified death" is not in itself an oxymoron. But death in the modern health care facility can be distinctly undignified. This is the main reason that, in spite of how painful it may be to do so, you should think about these issues before they ever become realities for you, your family and your caregivers. It is high time that the North American public, led by its medical workers, learned to regain respect for death not as the enemy but as the human event that it is.

# 11 The Emergency Room

Even if you set to work right away to consider the options discussed in the last chapter or to draft your advance directive, an accident or sudden illness could bring matters to a head at any moment. If you have the misfortune to face tough choices for yourself or a family member amid the hubbub and high emotional pitch of an emergency room, you'll find it's a world apart from making calm, informed decisions in the comfort of your home.

In 1978, an American doctor named Samuel Shem wrote a novel called *The House of God.* Irreverent in its portrayal of modern hospital medicine, it was popular reading among the medical and nursing staffs at many North American hospitals at the time. One of the reasons for its popularity was that it put into print the frustrated, burned-out feelings of many an overworked, jaded intern. One particularly jarring term Shem uses is "GOMER," which Shem spells out as "Get Out of My Emergency Room." Shem further defines a GOMER as "a human being who has lost — often through age — what goes into being a human being": a frightening commentary on the lack of respect that emergency health care personnel may have for aging people.

Obviously, not everyone in health care shares this attitude, but the term or similarly disrespectful ones are used by too many people in too many real hospitals. It is the manifestation of some of the deep-seated, often subconscious feelings that medical personnel who are trained to deal with crises have about aging patients or those they feel they can do nothing for. Their approach to medical care can differ from that of workers in other parts of the hospital. To ensure you get the emergency care you want, it helps to understand the perspective of the emergency team and the context in which they work.

## THE CRITICAL MOMENT

Even if you have yet to experience a health crisis, you've seen them on television. They are dramatic, baffling and above all, emotionally stressful for everyone involved.

It could happen to you. Say you have been admitted to hospital following a car accident in which you were severely injured. At sixty-eight, you also have terminal cancer, and you have recently been told that you probably only have about six months to live. You are in a great deal of pain and it is evident that you have internal injuries. The surgeon called to the emergency department tells you that you need immediate surgery to uncover the exact location of the internal bleeding and to stop it, or you will hemorrhage to death. You are conscious and coherent right now, capable of making such a decision for yourself, but as you continue to bleed you will lose consciousness. At the moment, it looks like you could die today or tomorrow in relative comfort, or six months from now in pain. If you are to make the decision yourself, it can't wait.

Or perhaps your seventy-six-year-old father has just suffered what appeared to be a cardiac arrest while he was out shopping. A bystander applied CPR and revived him, and an ambulance brought him to the nearest emergency room. He would be dead now if a well-meaning stranger had not acted, but he has not regained consciousness. The cardiologist comes to you and says that your father is suffering from a cardiac arrhythmia (a problem with the electrical conduction system in his heart), which originally caused his heart to stop beating. If he does not have emergency surgery to implant a pacemaker, he will die. He needs a decision.

To you, these are shocking, unexpected and frightening events. To the emergency medical personnel, they constitute a normal day at the office. Keep this in mind as you wonder why everyone around you can keep functioning while you face such agonizing choices.

## THE CAREGIVERS' PERSPECTIVE

When you are faced with a crisis, you need information and you need it fast. The people who will be most valuable to you in an emergency will often be the medical and nursing personnel assigned to care for you or your family member.

People who choose to work in fast-paced, high-stress medical situations are not like people who choose family medicine or geriatrics. These personal factors and value systems make them a different breed, and you need to make them your allies. This is not going to be easy, because you usually have a very short period of time in which to develop the relationship that is necessary.

Several factors affect how doctors and nurses deal with an emergency and thus also affect how they will interpret the events to you and what they will recommend as a decision.

## BELIEF IN A DUTY TO TREAT

There are many areas of ethical fuzziness in medicine and nursing, but one area that is clear is that emergency personnel have a duty to treat. Section 5 of the American Medical Association's Principles of Medical Ethics clearly says, "A physician may choose whom he will serve. In an emergency, however, he should render service to the best of his ability." Similarly, article 12 of the Canadian Medical Association's Code of Ethics states that the physician has the right to refuse to accept a patient "except in an emergency." In fact, in an emergency when consent cannot be obtained from you or your family, the duty to treat overrides your right to consent. The health professionals will treat first and ask questions later.

## FEAR OF LITIGATION

As consumers have become more knowledgeable about their health care over the past decade or two, the number of lawsuits against doctors and nurses has increased dramatically. The result is that health care workers are often gun-shy. They will do just about anything to avoid appearing negligent and being sued; they are only human and need to protect themselves. This attitude tends to result in both over-treatment and recommendations to patient and family to over-treat.

Keep in mind too that health care workers in emergencies rarely have long-term knowledge of their patients. They do not have the advantage of knowing your history, your beliefs or your wishes, as a family doctor with a fifteen-year relationship with the family would.

## EFFICIENCY AS AN OBJECTIVE

Although cure may not always be the appropriate goal in the treatment of older adults, acute care hospitals and emergency personnel are geared toward efficiency and "fixing" things. This attitude of efficiency and cure again results in treatment recommendations that may not take into consideration other factors, like family situations and chronic conditions.

## HOSPITAL POLICIES

Certain hospitals, notably those with religious affiliations, may have unqualified enthusiasm for preserving life by the use of all available medical means. You may feel subtle but clear pressures to agree to this approach. If it does mirror your own feelings, then you are not at a disadvantage; but a mismatch between your views and the hospital's could add to the difficulty of your decision. Look into the policies of the facilities where you might end up in an emergency so that you can choose a hospital that shares your point of view, if at all possible.

## TECHNOLOGY

The rapid growth of medical knowledge and the ongoing development of equipment makes it difficult for any single medical practitioner to be sure that he or she possesses all the facts at a given time, unless all possible diagnostic avenues have been followed. Even then no one can be 100 percent sure of a prognosis. Therefore, in an emergency, doctors may buy time by suggesting that a vital support system be used until the situation is clearer. Once these life supports are started, it can be extremely difficult to discontinue them.

## YOUR RIGHTS IN
## AN EMERGENCY

Although your rights in an acute medical emergency are essentially the same as they are in other circumstances, in the heat of the moment, some of them may be forgotten by either you or the medical personnel you are dealing with. It is even more important at a time like this to think about your rights, as the result of neglecting them can be disastrous.

First, you have a *right to be treated*. This is generally not a problem in an emergency. The ethical and technological bent of most health care workers in these areas is such that they will, as mentioned before, tend to treat first and ask questions later if left to their own devices. In fact, you are more likely to be over-treated than under-treated.

You have a *right to be informed*, which can certainly be difficult in a crisis. First, you do not know who to ask or whose opinion to trust. Your best bet is probably to ask everyone, and gather as many different perspectives as possible. Second, health care workers may be so involved with treating you that the niceties, such as telling you or your family what they are doing or even who they are, might get lost in the battle. Finally, your own emotional state will be sure to have a significant effect on what you understand — or misunderstand — from the information that you do manage to glean. So both you and the health care team may be to blame if your right to be informed seems to be overlooked.

You still have a *right to give consent* if at all possible. But when a medical question needs an immediate answer and you are unable and your family are not available to give consent, you may be treated without that consent. Although medical personnel have an obligation to find someone who can give consent, this may not be realistically possible. If you *are* able to give consent, don't sign anything you don't understand.

Rights are only useful insofar as they can be exercised. Time constraints in an emergency may prevent you from properly exercising these rights as you would wish. Thinking about these issues in advance will give you at least a chance of making better decisions.

## DEALING WITH THE FALLOUT

The decisions you make will have a variety of effects, on those around you as well as yourself.

To go back to the scenarios described earlier, what decision would you make if you were the sixty-eight-year-old with internal bleeding and terminal cancer? Whatever decision you make, you and those close to you will have to live with it. Perhaps you are overwhelmed by the emotion of the moment; with your granddaughter standing outside the room, you decide that you want to go to her wedding. If you allow the doctor to perform surgery and, in spite of the medical staff's best efforts, you do not immediately improve, your consent will have given them reason to believe that they should be even more aggressive with their treatment. If you do improve and live to attend the event, you may have to suffer in the end with your cancer, and you may find it much more difficult to find someone who will allow you to be "snowed" to your final resting place by increasing doses of painkillers.

On the other hand, if you refuse treatment and you and your family have never discussed these issues before, you may leave behind a very confused family. This confusion may even turn into anger at you and at what you have done to them, because they may not understand your decision and you may not have had time to explain it to them.

The bottom line in crisis decision-making — in health care as in other fields — is that if you have to make a quick decision about an issue you have never considered before, you may not like the results. It

takes great effort to separate cool, clear-headed thinking from the emotions that usually accompany these
unforeseen situations. The more you plan in advance
and the more you and your family understand about
your own and one another's attitudes toward health
care as you age, the easier it will be to live with the
decisions that you make in a medical emergency.

# 12 : Lifeboats for All?

I<small>T HAD BEEN A</small> relatively quiet Sunday night in the emergency room of the City Hospital. Young Bill Greenberg, the on-duty emergency room physician, was having his second cup of coffee and discussing the hockey game with one of the interns in the lounge when the charge nurse popped her head in the door and said, "Two cardiacs on the way. Better hop to it."

Dr. Greenberg took a last gulp from his coffee, rinsed the cup out at the sink and grabbed his stethoscope on the way out the door. He was thinking that it never rains but it pours. Two patients with heart attacks at the same time, and the cardiology resident was tied up in the coronary care unit. Well, he would have to get by the best he could on his own.

As he headed toward the ambulance bays, the automatic doors swung open and the medics rushed in with a stretcher at full speed. They were just beginning to give their first information about the patient when, not thirty seconds later, the other set of doors opened and the second heart patient was wheeled into the foyer. It was very difficult to hear

179

what anyone was saying. Dr. Greenberg followed the first stretcher into the cardiac room and directed the nurse to get him the information about the second.

When the stories were finally sorted out and the patients were stabilized, the following stories emerged. The first patient through the doors was a seventy-year-old man with a massive heart attack. He was stabilized but would need intensive cardiac care for best recovery. The second patient through the doors was a thirty-seven-year-old woman with exactly the same story. She had now been stabilized following a massive heart attack but would also need intensive cardiac care for best recovery.

Dr. Greenberg had a problem on this night in the emergency room: there was only one bed in the cardiac care unit. It was up to him to decide who would get it.

Scenes like this, requiring allocation of scarce resources, happen every day in hospitals all across North America, and with the health care cost crunch they are likely to become more frequent. The decisions that are made are based on everything from hospital policy to the golden rule.

Although no one can put a dollar value on human life, it is surely valid, even responsible, to consider how expensive it is to die under modern medical care. When a life is coming to its natural end, you should give some thought to the costs of unnaturalness.

Of the close to $970 billion spent on health care annually in North America, almost 28 percent is spent on elderly people during the last days of their lives. Since as many as 90 percent of these people have never discussed their treatment wishes with their caregivers, that means as much as $244 billion is spent on dying patients who have not expressed a wish to be treated. If our countries had infinite amounts of money, this huge expense might not be missed. But, of course, we do not.

Money, materials and people are all in increasingly short supply in the health care systems in both the U.S. and Canada. Someone has to pay, and someone has to decide who gets what is paid for. These two someones are usually two different people, but they don't always have to be. Perhaps *you* who pay the bills (through either taxation or direct payment to private insurers) could decide what you should take from the system. As a final aspect of exerting power over your own health care decisions as you age, we are going to suggest that you consider not only your own good, but also the good of others. We are going to ask you to think about something that perhaps no one has ever suggested to you before. We are going to suggest that, when the time comes for a decision about who will receive treatment and who will not, you may be able to decide to give up your place in the lifeboat.

## WOMEN AND CHILDREN FIRST?

The North American public has an insatiable appetite for more and better high-tech medical "fixes." Just try telling someone about the new multimillion-dollar toy that your local hospital has just acquired. Either her eyes will light up at your luck in being

near such a well-equipped hospital, or she will immediately begin telling you about the newer, better and
more expensive gadget that her local hospital has just
bought. Neither of you is likely to know clearly just
what either piece of high-tech equipment is used for,
or who might conceivably benefit from it, but modern
medicine is only as good as its gadgets, isn't it?

Both the increasing age of our population and
high-technology medicine are among the top candidates for blame for increasing health care costs. The
place where these two currently meet is at the end of
life. Whatever the reasons for the costs, they are a
fact of life and we, as individuals, should consider
what part we might play in helping health care professionals to decide how best to divide up the
resources that remain.

The health care systems in North America have
been likened to a sinking ship. When all the passengers have been summoned on deck with their life
preservers, it is found that there are not enough
lifeboats to go around. There used to be an old adage
that women and children were to be saved first, but
with the modern view that ethics is situational, this
once-accepted guide to action is no longer taken for
granted. In modern medicine, the principles of fairness are generally believed to be unbiased as to age
or gender. How, then, can we be fair about giving out
the lifeboat seats? This is the problem faced by those
concerned about the principle of justice in health care
resource allocation.

Two authors of a now classic textbook on medical
ethics have been telling health profession students for

over a decade that there are five traditional approaches that might possibly be used to make sure that decisions about who gets what are fair and just. The principle of women and children first is not among them. They have suggested that we might give people their share based on:

■ equal division of whatever is in scarce supply;

■ their level of need;

■ how much effort they put into obtaining what they want;

■ how much they have contributed to society;

■ their value to society now and in the future.

As you might imagine, these are not easy to apply, nor are they considered fair by everyone. For example, the following questions have not been answered: How do you measure a person's value to society? Is it by past contributions, future contributions, gender, race, age? Upon what do you base the measurement of medical need? What do you do if you decide that two people have an equal need, but both cannot be treated?

Other principles have been suggested. These include giving care to people based on:

■ the ability to pay;

■ their place in line (first come, first served).

There are considerable arguments against giving to people only what they can pay for — although some people would contend that this is common practice — and the notion of taking a place in line is just as nasty a thought to some. Waiting for your turn would mean that even if your need is greater, you would have to wait in line behind those whose need was less but who were there first.

Here are two other possibilities. Perhaps we should give to each according to:

- chance (have a lottery);
- the likelihood of a good medical outcome.

Most of us are of the opinion that someone else always wins the lottery. And a good outcome may be very difficult to predict. Furthermore, should the measurement of that outcome be based on quality or quantity of life, and who will make the decision and referee any conflicts?

In practice, doctors rely on varying sets of guidelines to make their decisions. These include:

- their own personal beliefs and values that they grew up with;
- the opinions of their colleagues, which they seek out in difficult situations;
- what they believe is included in the code of ethics of their professional association;
- hospital policies and procedures.

As you can see, the decisions about who should get what are extremely complex. But choosing by medical outcome begins to ring the bells of fairness and justice for many health professionals and non-health professionals alike. By its very nature, however, it has implications for older adults, since many medical approaches are likely to have poorer outcomes as we age. Does this mean that we should be discriminated against because of our age?

## OLDER ADULTS: DEFINING THEIR SHARE

There are many different ways to view the idea of aging. Sometimes how you see it depends upon whether you consider yourself among the aging or not. Whatever view you hold and whatever view is most common in society, however, will be certain to have an impact on how you define your share of what is available in health care resources.

One medical writer has an interesting way of defining the continuum of society's views about the aged. She places these views on a scale, from the most negative to the most positive:

- Aging is the direct opposite of health and vitality. This, the most negative view of aging, holds that being healthy and being old are incompatible.

- Although aging in itself may not be such a bad thing, seeing it in others reminds us that we are mortal.

- Although the aged are really of no value to society, they should be protected because they cannot protect themselves.

- Aging is a distinctive human experience, and it is therefore worthy, at the very least, of both the medical researcher's and the medical practitioner's time.

■ Elderly people are to be cherished by society for their wisdom and their past accomplishments. This, of course, is the most positive view of aging, but it is not currently the most widespread attitude in North America, unfortunately.

As you can see, it is highly likely that if one of these views of aging overshadows the others in a particular society, it is likely to have an effect on what share of scarce health resources is made available to you as you age. If aging is considered to be the antithesis of health anyway, why would physicians even consider treating the older adult with anything more vigorous than comfort measures?

It is true, however, in many cases, that the older the individual, the poorer his or her general health. With poorer general health comes the likelihood that medical treatment will not be as successful as it would be in a younger person. This plain reality is often mistaken for ageism in health care.

## THE POWER TO DEFINE YOUR OWN SHARE

Throughout this book we have stressed exercising your personal autonomy, your right to make your own decisions. It may seem to you now that these decisions will often be out of your hands. This can be true, but it doesn't have to be that way.

One of the final decisions that you will have to make in your life is deciding when enough is enough. When your life's story is drawing to a close and your life's plan is fulfilled, you might refrain from asking what the health care system can do for you and ask instead what you can do for the health care system and society. Consider too that your children and grandchildren are a part of that society. Paradoxical as it may seem for those of us who are a part of the so-called "me generation," a decision to stop fighting death may just be our ultimate expression of autonomy and free choice.

Not everyone will want to step aside. It is, however, a concept worth considering and worth talking over with your loved ones before you have to make it. A society and culture that allowed many healthy young men to sacrifice their lives for their countries on numerous battlefields through the years should just as surely respect those who give of themselves at the end of their days so that others may live better lives.

Clearly, the best time to make decisions is when we are fully capable of doing it for ourselves. These decisions should be respected. If we also respected the rights of others when we made those decisions, what a great world it would be. Perhaps respect is, after all, the best of all possible guiding principles.

# For More Information

## Books of Interest

Beinfield, Harriet and Efrem Korngold. *Between Heaven and Earth: A Guide to Chinese Medicine.* New York: Ballantine Books, 1991.

Callahan, Daniel. *Setting Limits: Medical Goals in an Aging Society.* New York: Simon and Schuster, 1987.

Callahan, Daniel. *What Kind of Life: The Limits of Medical Progress.* New York: Simon and Schuster, 1990.

Fish, Sharon. *Alzheimer's: Caring for Your Loved One, Caring for Yourself.* Batavia, Ill.: Lion Publishing, 1990.

Hatfield, Bob and Bruce Hatfield. *Matters of Life and Death.* Winfield, B.C.: Wood Lake Books, 1985.

Humphry, Derek. *Dying With Dignity: Understanding Euthanasia.* Secausus, N.J.: Carol Publishing Group, 1992.

189

Humphry, Derek. *Final Exit: The Practicalities of Self-Deliverance and Assisted Suicide for the Dying.* Secausus, N.J.: Hemlock Society, 1991.

Inlander, Charles B. and Eugene I. Pavalon. *Your Medical Rights.* Boston: Little Brown, 1990.
Mace, Nancy. *The 36-Hour Day: A Family Guide to Caring for Persons with Alzheimer's Disease.* Baltimore: Johns Hopkins University Press, 1991.

Molloy, William. *Vital Choices: Life, Death and the Health Care Crisis.* Toronto: Viking, 1993.

Molloy, William and Virginia Mepham. *Let Me Decide: The Health Care Directive That Speaks for You When You Can't.* Toronto: Penguin, 1989.

Moore, Pat with Charles Paul Conn. *Disguised: A True Story.* Waco, Texas: Word Books, 1985.

Radey, Charles. *Choosing Wisely: How Patients and Their Families Can Make the Right Decisions About Life and Death.* New York: Doubleday, 1992.

Rollin, Betty. *Last Wish.* New York: Simon and Schuster, 1985.

University of Toronto Centre for Bioethics Living Will – a form and explanatory notes available for C$5.00, including postage and GST, from the University of Toronto Centre for Bioethics, 88 College Street, Toronto, Ont. M5G 1L4. Tel: 416-978-2709; fax: 416-978-1911. Bulk prices are also available.

## Organizations of Interest

We have selected a number of national organizations that can provide information or support. In addition, there are likely to be local groups within your own community. Inquire at a volunteer center or public library.

## CANADA

**Canadian Association of Retired Persons**
27 Queen Street E., Suite 1304
Toronto, Ontario
M5C 2M6
416-363-8748

This association is a non-profit national organization founded to improve the quality of life for Canadians over the age of fifty. Membership is open. It publishes a newspaper for members on a quarterly basis.

**Dying with Dignity: A Canadian Society Concerned with the Quality of Dying**
600 Eglinton Avenue E., Suite 401
Toronto, Ontario
M4P 1P3
416-486-3998

This organization was formed to educate people about issues related to death and dying. It distributes a quarterly newsletter, *Living Will*, to its members and supports the recognition of voluntary euthanasia.

**One Voice — The Canadian Seniors Network**
1005 — 350 Sparks Street
Ottawa, Ontario
K1R 7S8
613-238-7624

A non-profit organization of seniors working together to make Canada a better place to age, this network facilitates research, education and government lobbying on all aspects of aging. Among other publications, it produces a newsletter four times a year.

**National Advisory Council on Aging**
Government of Canada
473 Albert Street
Ottawa, Ontario
K1A 0K9
613-957-1968

One of the most useful things that this federal government agency does is act as a clearinghouse for organizations of interest to older adults and their families. Its database can provide lists of regional and national organizations.

**Patients' Rights Association**
40 Homewood Avenue, Suite 315
Toronto, Ontario
M4Y 2K2
416-923-9629

Primarily devoted to consumer issues in health care, this association publishes a newsletter, *The Patient Advocate*, a handbook of patients' rights and a variety of brochures on related issues.

## UNITED STATES

**Gray Panthers**
1424 16th Street NW, Suite 602
Washington, DC
20036
202-387-3111

With 7,000 members, the Gray Panthers is a consciousness-raising group of older adults and young people whose main objective is to combat ageism. It also conducts research and seminars on age-related issues and publishes *Gray Panther Network*, a quarterly newspaper, and *Gray Panther Washington Watch*, a bimonthly.

**National Alliance of Senior Citizens**
1700 18th Street NW, Suite 401
Washington, DC
20009
202-986-0117

Representing the views of senior citizens before Congress and state legislatures, the alliance has 100,000 members. It maintains a library for political and general research, conducts educational programs and publishes *Senior Guardian* monthly.

**National Council of Senior Citizens**
1331 F Street NW
Washington, DC
20004-1171
202-347-8800

With 5 million members, this national council is an organization of senior citizens' clubs, associations and councils whose main purposes are education and action to maintain Medicare and social security, the enactment of a national health plan including long-term care, and reduced costs of drugs. Among other things, it sponsors rallies and educational workshops, provides speakers and maintains a library. It produces two monthly publications: *Retirement Newsletter* and *Senior Citizens News*.

## National Council on the Aging
409 3rd Street SW, No. 200
Washington, DC
20024
202-479-6665

Membership in this council is diverse, including individuals in business and industry, organized labor and the health professions, social workers, librarians, clergy and educators. The council works to promote concern for older people and to develop methods and resources to meet their needs. It maintains a 12,000-volume library and conducts research and demonstration programs. It publishes a quarterly volume that abstracts books and articles on aging, health care and retirement issues; a bimonthly tabloid, *NCOA Networks*; and a bimonthly magazine, *Perspective on Aging*, which is available to members only.

## Mature Outlook
6001 N. Clark Street
Chicago, IL
60660
800-336-6330

Some 800,000 members strong, this organization bills itself as a for-profit venture that provides benefits, services and information to its members who are over age fifty. Publishes *Mature Outlook Magazine* and *Mature Outlook Newsletter*.

**National Caucus and Center on Black Aged**
1424 K St. NW, Suite 500
Washington, DC
20005
202-637-8400

This national organization seeks to improve living conditions primarily for low-income, elderly black Americans by advocating changes in federal and state laws. In addition, it promotes community awareness of problems and issues of older blacks, and operates an employment program in fourteen states. It publishes a quarterly newsletter, *Golden Page*.